Between
the
Dying
the
Dead

Terrace Books, a division of the University of Wisconsin Press, takes its name from the Memorial Union Terrace, located at the University of Wisconsin–Madison. Since its inception in 1907, the Wisconsin Union has provided a venue for students, faculty, staff, and alumni to debate art, music, politics, and the issues of the day. It is a place where theater, music, drama, dance, outdoor activities, and major speakers are made available to the campus and the community. To learn more about the Union, visit www.union.wisc.edu.

Between
the Dying
and the Dead

Dr. Jack Kevorkian's Life
and the Battle to
Legalize Euthanasia

Neal Nicol and
Harry Wylie

The University of Wisconsin Press
Terrace Books

The University of Wisconsin Press
1930 Monroe Street
Madison, Wisconsin 53711

www.wisc.edu/wisconsinpress/

2   4   5   3   1

Cover photo: Amy Powers
Cover and text design by ok?design
Printed and bound in the United Kingdom by Mackays of Chatham Ltd.,
Chatham, Kent

Library of Congress Cataloging-in-Publication Data

Nicol, Neal.
Between the dying and the dead: Dr. Jack Kevorkian's life
and the battle to legalize euthanasia /
Neal Nicol and Harry Wilie.
p. cm.
ISBN 0-299-21710-8 (hardcover : alk. paper)
1. Kevorkian, Jack. 2. Terminally ill. 3. Pathologists–United States–Biography.
4. Right to die. 5. Assisted suicide. I. Wilie, Harry. II. Title.
III. Title: Dr. Jack Kevorkian's life and the battle to legalize euthanasia.
[DNLM: 1. Kevorkian, Jack. 2. Physicians–United States–Biography.
3. Euthanasia–legislation & jurisprudence–United States.
WZ 100 K43n 2006]
R726.N53   2006
179.7–dc22   2006006903

First published in the United Kingdom in 2006 by Vision,
a division of Satin Publications Ltd.
www.visionpaperbacks.co.uk

Few men are willing to brave the disapproval of their fellows, the censure of their colleagues, the wrath of society. Moral courage is a rarer commodity than bravery in battle or great intelligence. Yet it is the one essential, vital quality for those that seek to change a world that yields most painfully to change.

Robert Kennedy

CONTENTS

ACKNOWLEDGEMENTS

This book couldn't be without Dr Jack Kevorkian – his work, his dedication and of course his blessing. Others have contributed immensely, we trust we have omitted no one and we list alphabetically: Doug Conciatu, Mary Cuddihy, Jim Dean, Geoffrey Fieger, Vanig Godoshian, Ray Good, Ruth Holmes, Sharyn Kolberg, Norbert Lakemaker, Jack Lessenberry, Dr Stan Levy, Gary Lind-Sinanian, Dr Jack Lynch, Mayer Morganroth, Fuensanta Plaza, Brian Russell, Bob Ryeson, Diane Ryeson, Gene Ryeson, Michael Schwartz and Melody Youk.

Preface

We were visiting Prisoner # 284797 at Michigan's Thumb Correctional Facility. We had been travelling to see Jack at six prisons over the previous five years, usually on a monthly basis where we stayed for about five hours; we wanted him to be free of his cell for as long as possible. Other prisoners with family and friends would look disparagingly at our coffee table because we were either in heated argument or uproarious laughter. We were sometimes rebuked by the guards, but generally they left us alone, perhaps appreciating a change to the typical dour composure of inmates and guests.

The level of banter this particular day was no different from others. It is difficult to describe the joy of jousting verbally with a person like Dr Jack Kevorkian. The conversation may have started about a comment on the Iraq conflagration which reminded someone about *All Quiet on The Western Front* with Lew Ayres, which brought to mind Mae West that bounced off to World War II life preservers, and perhaps breast implants and then general chemical breakthroughs and Germany's dominance in chemistry, perhaps Austria, which reminded someone of Freud and his contribution to modern psychiatry, perhaps Jung – it was always thus; wonderful!

Jack has had much published, from serious papers in medical journals to not so serious medical books like *Slimericks*, a diet book by Limerick format. We asked Jack why he never wrote his biography, especially now that he had some time on his hands, and he said that Neal had all the information and requested he carry out the task. Neal deferred the research and composition to me, and a partnership was established.

We hope this biography illustrates that the abrasive persona he put forth to the public is not the real Jack Kevorkian. Jack is brilliant, eccentric and self-deprecating. He is tremendously witty and great fun to be with. He is an artist, a musician, a composer, a linguist and a philosopher. And he has personally helped many individuals end their suffering and changed the way society thinks about dying.

Few people know that he was sentenced, for all intents and purposes, to life in prison. Many believe him dead. The institution called Legislative America has so isolated him from the public that, by disallowing media contact and legal appeals, they have succeeded in their goal of shutting him in and shutting him up – out of sight, out of mind. Jack is a remarkable human being, whose life and work deserve to be celebrated. We hope *Between the Dying and the Dead* will educate the world to the plight of this humanitarian.

Harry Wylie

Chapter 1

THE CRUCIBLE

To many of those who have known him personally, he is a saint and a saviour. To many of those who only know of him, he is the worst kind of sinner. Millions of people around the world know the name Dr Jack Kevorkian, but few know anything about the man. When his fight to legalise euthanasia was making headlines in the 1990s, the public saw only the macabre 'Dr Death' – the often abrasive, always outspoken proponent of the right of the terminally ill to end their suffering on their own terms. But behind that persona lies a complicated man with a compelling story. He was a former child prodigy, the son of Armenian refugees who came to America to escape the Turkish genocide. Starting with nothing, his parents soon found themselves raising a precocious student, a boy his less-gifted teachers dreaded but whom the neighbourhood kids idolised. His early talents ranged from woodwork to linguistics to science experiments in the basement. Later, he became a brilliant pathologist, devoting his life to the unusual pursuit of extracting social benefit from death.

Dr Kevorkian's passion brought him into constant conflict with the society that he saw himself as trying to help. At every step along the way, he went at loggerheads with people who were not ready for his ideas. He did not just take on the medical establishment and the law; throughout his life he dared to challenge a taboo as old as human civilisation – the taboo against death. He dared to suggest that we treat dying, suffering and suicide rationally.

Jack Kevorkian is a complex individual, full of fascinating contradictions. He is outspoken, brash, egotistical and intensely committed to the causes in which he believes. He is also a shy, eccentric man who lived a monastic, ethical life, buying his clothes at the Salvation Army and subsisting on the plainest of food, particularly white bread. He lacks the capacity to lie so much that when he played poker with his friends he never bluffed, and if he bet, everyone folded.

Regardless of how one feels about his politics, Dr Kevorkian changed the way most of us think about dying. Because of him, we now have living wills and the right to refuse resuscitation. A November 2005 poll by the Pew Research Center showed that 29 per cent of the people surveyed have living wills – more than twice the number who had them in 1990. Attitudes towards pain management for terminally ill patients have changed dramatically. Rather than being withheld necessary medication in case they become addicted, many patients are now given the ability, through implanted pumps, to self-control the dose of pain medication they receive. And the number of doctors who admit to quietly complying with a patient's request for a lethal dose of medication is steadily rising.

None of these changes came without a fight.

By 1999, Dr Jack Kevorkian had become the well-known poster boy for assisted suicide, the infamous Dr Death of headline

news. He had made headlines by evading prosecution countless times. Physician-assisted suicide had even been made legal
in Oregon, and 86 per cent of the country supported its being
made legal nationwide. Through the controversy he generated,
he made dying with dignity part of the popular consciousness.
But the movement was stagnating, in part because prosecutors
had become reluctant to try Kevorkian under new laws against
assisted suicide for fear that he might win in the Supreme Court
and have the laws struck down. They hoped to wait him out, let
his popularity die down as he got older and America quickly
forgot him. So Kevorkian decided to force the law's hand with a
case that no one would be able to ignore – a case of a terminally
ill patient who had lost so many of his faculties that he would
be unable to work Kevorkian's suicide machine, requiring the
doctor to administer the lethal injection himself. He would videotape the suicide – or medicide, as he called it – and send the tape
to the media, appear on national television and dare the state to
come after him.

Tom Youk was a shy lumberjack of a man with thick curly brown
hair who worked hard throughout his life, from delivering papers
as a young boy, then labouring as a chef's assistant and as a hospital orderly as a young adult. When the Air Force drafted him in
1966 he was considering becoming an auto mechanic.

A decorated sergeant in Germany, when he returned to America in 1969 Tom decided to go to college on the GI Bill and
graduated with an accounting degree in 1974. He met his wife,
Melody, in the mid 70s at a high school reunion. Later in life,
when accounting started to tire him, he struck out on his own. A
25-year member of the Porsche Club of America, he had always

3

loved mechanical work, so he turned his hobby of restoring vintage cars into a business, Vintage 356 Haus. He and his company flourished, and soon he was living out a fantasy, nursing dottering old 356 and 911 Porsches that everyone had given up on into growling, roaring racing machines. He even retooled a 1965 Porsche and began racing it at the age of 50, whipping younger drivers on local tracks. He toured the amateur circuit and finally, in 1996, he became the Ohio Valley champion. It seemed like nothing was impossible.

Then in June that year, Tom was diagnosed with amyotrophic lateral sclerosis (ALS), Lou Gehrig's disease. ALS is a progressive neuromuscular disorder caused by the death of the motor nerve cells that control voluntary muscle movement. Tom soon discovered that he was facing an unwinnable race. There was no cure for ALS. He had, if he was lucky, three to five years to live. The path to his inevitable death wouldn't be an easy one. His muscles would slowly stop responding. At first he might find it hard to walk. Then his hands would stop working. His tongue and jaw would become uncontrollable. He would drool. He would choke on his own spit. His faeces would have to be scooped from his bowels. He wouldn't be able to move or to talk, and soon it would become hard to breathe. And through it all, his mind would be alive. He would know what was happening. He would be a prisoner in his own body without hope of parole.

He tried to fight it. He visited every doctor who offered a glimmer of hope, but the best they had was increasingly ineffective pain medication; medication which they limited, as the medical establishment dictated, fearing turning him into a drug addict. They told him to be brave. So Tom tried to fight ALS with the same analytic, determined approach he had used throughout his life, researching new information, seeking alternative treatments as well as participating in experimental drug therapies through the University of Michigan Hospital.

Tom Youk didn't give up easily. He soon found that he couldn't work the clutch on his racecar, so he modified it so that his hands could do the work his feet once did. Then his arms stopped working. Within a few months only the thumb and first two fingers on his right hand moved, and speaking took his full concentration. In spite of the doctors' best efforts, he had trouble swallowing. His own body slowly began to strangle him. He had a food tube put directly into his stomach in late August, 1998, but his body wouldn't metabolise the food. Nothing could help him breathe and his lung capacity dropped to 25 per cent of normal. He didn't want to live totally paralysed, unable to speak, relying on machines and others for everything. He didn't want to fight through days of pain, waiting for his body to finally decide to kill him.

One day he told his brother Terry that the agony was like having his body plugged into an electric socket. It was the kind of pain that medicine couldn't help. 'I don't want to die,' Tom said, 'but I don't want to live like this either.' He asked his doctors if they would help him commit suicide. He explained that he didn't want to wait in pain, in constant panic when his body choked him, or when his lungs forgot to breathe. He wanted to pick the time and place of his death, to say goodbye with his family around him, to die with dignity. The doctors wouldn't help him; their interpretation of the Hippocratic oath forbade them. Doctors train to fight death to the end and a doctor that actually caused death they deemed a traitor to their profession. Tom's request dismayed the doctors who were unwilling to accept that they couldn't do anything for him. Others pointed out religious concerns; the Church said he would end up in hell if he committed suicide. While several doctors sympathised, they considered their hands tied. If they helped him, they could lose their medical licences. The best they could do was give him more pain medication (mostly to relieve his anxiety rather than to reduce the pain) and tell him to be strong.

The Youk family contacted the Hemlock Society who recommended the hoarding of medication to die by overdose or placing a plastic bag over the head for suffocation, or both. The pain and suffering Tom would have to endure whilst hoarding medication was unthinkable, and death by baggy the family deemed barbaric.

Tom knew of one doctor who would help, and he asked his family to contact Dr Jack Kevorkian. They resisted, but he convinced them that death – on his terms – really was what he wanted. He was the one suffering, and it would be an act of cruelty to force him to keep living.

They found Dr Kevorkian's address on the internet. Though Tom could barely speak, he dictated his letter to Melody and Terry. They sent the letter by overnight mail, and the next day Jack called them. He needed to see Tom's medical records. He wanted to make sure that Tom had done everything the traditional medical establishment suggested for treating his disease and easing the pain. Tom's family sent another overnight package, this one bursting with all of Tom's medical files. Four days later Jack called them to say he would visit them soon. He wanted to talk to Tom.

Dr Kevorkian exercised care in selecting his patients. He received letters continuously – from the old and lonely, depressed by their isolation but otherwise healthy, to eccentrics claiming agonising pain because of constipation, obesity or fantasies that malicious aliens had invaded their bodies. He also turned down numerous requests from disgruntled children afraid of losing inheritances due to their mother's love affairs with Las Vegas slot machines.

Dr Kevorkian chose his patients carefully, first and foremost because of his personal convictions, but also because he knew his enemies were waiting for him to make a mistake.

By that summer of 1998, he had been brought up on charges by the state of Michigan eight times. Each time he was acquitted, the charges were dropped or a mistrial was declared. The medical establishment also tried to prevent Jack's work. Michigan state medical regulators had suspended Kevorkian's medical licence in 1991. But when they issued him an order to cease and desist from practising medicine he publicly burned it. In 1993, the state of California – the only other state in which he was licensed to practise medicine – also suspended his licence. His involvement with assisted suicide incensed the America Medical Association (AMA), and they denounced him as a danger to society. In response, Kevorkian filed a $10 million defamation suit against the Michigan State Medical Society and the AMA, alleging that the two organisations libelled him in a November 1995 AMA press release that called him 'a reckless instrument of death' who 'poses a great threat to the public'. The suit was dismissed by a Michigan appeals court in August 1999, saying that the statements were 'protected opinion'.

In turn, Kevorkian claimed the medical establishment was corrupt. He had long retired from practising pathology in hospitals. He felt that money was more important to most doctors than easing pain and suffering. It also infuriated him when doctors began using religious arguments on the sanctity of life as a basis for denying him his licence.

Despite his personal views, Kevorkian had support from many churches, especially Presbyterian and Unitarian churches who opened their doors to many of his supporters. One Unitarian minister even requested of his superiors that he – and others who might want help – be allowed to have his own assisted suicide in the church. (He was turned down.)

Though Kevorkian understood that people might look to religious institutions for comfort at times of death, and encouraged patients to use the counsel of religious advisors, he considered all talk of an afterlife juvenile. When a person died, the body solely succumbed to natural decay. There was nothing else. Kevorkian felt assisting in someone's suicide was a medical procedure no different than amputating a leg. It was a tough thing for a doctor to do, but it was sometimes necessary. In fact, Kevorkian believed doctors shouldn't feel they were helping end someone's life, but that they were ending someone's suffering. Since not every doctor could be that detached, Kevorkian argued that it needed to be a specialty in its own right. He envisioned gathering other doctors like himself and training them in a new specialty, obitiatry. His goal was to have government sanctioned national clinics – judicially bound and medically operated – to administer to the physically disenfranchised until they could be trusted to be objective when it came to deciding whether to assist in ending a patient's life.

As he planned for a future where numerous doctors assisted in 'medicide', he had realised that he needed to establish guidelines for the process in order to eliminate criticism. His developed doctrine stated that the patient had to clearly express a wish to die, and the family and outside psychiatrists had to be consulted in order to ensure that the choice wasn't due to depression or family pressure. The attending specialist had to review the patient's medical history to assure all possible alternatives had been explored and they had to perform the service for free, in order to prevent unscrupulous behaviour. Legal and secular counsel was strongly recommended. Finally, the doctor had to give the patient at least a month to consider their decision. He published his list of rules, passing it on to other doctors, which gained him both support and controversy. In the Tom Youk case, skirting his own rules haunted him in court.

When Dr Kevorkian finally reached the Youk home on September 16th, 1998, Melody Youk was surprised to find that Jack Kevorkian was not the man she had seen on television. He was quiet and calm, respectfully removing his hat as soon as he entered the house.

Tom Youk sat in a wheelchair in the living room. Jack Kevorkian introduced himself and his friend and helper Neal Nicol, and then, after asking permission, set up a video camera to tape their meeting. Tom was listless, but not in obvious agony. He struggled to swallow, and in that moment Kevorkian noticed the pain in Tom's eyes.

Kevorkian would later say, 'He just was terrified of choking to death, and he must have felt that he was on the verge of it. And I couldn't have him suffer in that kind of frame of mind because if a man is terrified, it's up to me to dispel that terror.'

Kevorkian took Tom's hand gently in his own, and leaned toward him. Tom's body relaxed, a sad smile flickered across his face. Kevorkian asked him to talk about his disease and what it had done to him. Tom paused, and then explained with great difficulty that his troubles began in 1994 after a knee operation (he modified his Porsche to operate the clutch with his hands so that he could keep racing for two more years) and that by 1997 he was in a wheelchair. The videotape shows Tom struggling to form the words and make himself heard. Jack had trouble understanding him. Finally, Melody interceded and translated for Tom, as she was one of the few people who could understand him.

'Can you move your legs at all?' Kevorkian asked.

'No.'

'How about your left arm?'

'No.'

'Try it,' Kevorkian pleaded. There was no movement. Tom was able to twitch the thumb on his right hand. 'That's all you can do?'

'Yes.'

Kevorkian motioned to the armrest of the wheelchair. 'You can't lift your hand off the thing there?'

Tom sadly shook his head.

'Have you talked this over with your mother, your brother and your wife?' Kevorkian asked. 'I suppose they tell you they want you to go on, don't they?'

Tom's mouth laboured over the words before finally releasing them. 'No, they understand. It's my decision.'

At another point, Kevorkian asked, 'Tom, have you thought about this now, your request? Have you thought hard about it?'

'If I had use of my arms, I wouldn't be doing it,' Tom said.

Kevorkian had previously assisted others in their suicides through use of machines. With one machine the patient pushed a button, enabling a sedative to course through an IV into their body, followed soon after by a drug that would stop their heartbeat. The other machine had a gas mask connected to a carbon monoxide tank. The patient just had to pull a clip off the tube and release the gas. In both variations, the patient had control. They decided when they were ready to die. But Tom was worried. He didn't have enough control over his hands to push a button or remove a clip. So he asked Kevorkian if they could forgo the machine altogether. Would Dr Kevorkian directly inject him?

Kevorkian had been waiting for a patient to ask him this question. He decided he would make a statement to the public after he assisted Tom. He had won a number of court cases over his assistance in other patients' suicides, but in those cases the patients had used his machine. They had been directly responsible for their own passing. With Tom, however, Kevorkian would be the one directly ending his life, and he would have it on videotape. Jack could show it to the press, and when the inevitable court case came, and he won it, doctors would no longer fear doing what he did.

Kevorkian pulled out a consent form.

'OK. Now I'm going to read it to you, Tom, and I want you to understand – I want to make sure you understand it, you have to listen closely and stop me if you can't understand it.'

'Yes.'

'It reads this way. "I, Thomas Youk, the undersigned, entirely voluntarily, without any reservation, external persuasion, pressure or duress, and after prolonged and thorough deliberation, hereby consent to the following medical procedure of my own choosing." And that you have chosen direct injection, or what they call active euthanasia, "to be administered by a competent medical professional in order to end with certainty my intolerable and hopelessly incurable suffering". Did you understand all that?'

'Yes.'

He handed Tom a pen to sign the form.

Tom struggled with his hand, forcing the pen to scratch his name. He wanted there to be no doubt that this was his choice, and with a measure of vanity, he wanted his final signature to be elegant and powerful, a final reminder of the man he once was.

Kevorkian studied the form. 'That's a fine signature,' he said. 'Were you an artist?'

Tom made an attempt to laugh and shook his head. He shared a smile with Kevorkian. It was a moment of life in the face of death. He no longer had to worry about when or how he would die. He now knew, and there was a peace in knowing.

But Kevorkian wasn't going to assist Tom that day. He had to give him a chance to change his mind.

'You're sure you thought about this very well, now?' Kevorkian asked.

'Very much.'

'You don't want to wait another month or so?'

'No, I …'

'You want to wait a week? How about two weeks? Two weeks?'

Tom shook his head in frustration.

'One week? Can you wait one week?'

'Yeah.'

'All right, we'll stretch it out one week, OK? Let's not hurry into this.'

Tom nodded.

Kevorkian shook Tom's hand, gathered up his video equipment, and prepared to walk out the door. Melody touched him on the arm, and said thank you. She then asked Kevorkian what would happen when he 'was done'.

'I'll leave the body here,' he said.

On the drive home from the Youk house, Kevorkian considered the choice that Tom had made, a choice Kevorkian had helped others with over 130 times in the past eight years. It was a choice that had been unavailable to his mother, Satenig, a refugee from the Armenian holocaust. When his family had learned she was dying of cancer, they had begged her doctors to help her die, but none would help. His mother suffered greatly and died in terror.

Kevorkian returned home, and spent the evening listening to a flute concerto.

Terry Youk called the next afternoon to say that Tom wanted it done 'now'. Kevorkian said he would do it, but that he didn't want Terry or Melody there. If the police were to come, he didn't want the two of them to have to face criminal charges.

'Would they really do that?' Terry asked.

'They think I'm a murderer,' Jack replied. 'They'll call you accomplices.'

When Kevorkian arrived, he found the door of the Youk house unlocked. He walked to Tom Youk's bedroom. Tom waited for him, propped up in bed. He gave a weak smile to the doctor. Dr Kevorkian, alone this time, again set up his video equipment.

'Are you sure you want to go ahead now?' Kevorkian asked.

Tom nodded. Dr Kevorkian methodically unpacked his equipment. He readied the appropriate solutions, then stepped over to Tom. He attached an EKG to Tom in order to measure heart rate. The IV would have to go into the veins on the back of Tom's hand.

'All right. I'm going to have you sign your name again and I'm ... and we're going to date it today, OK?'

Tom struggled with the form, and so Dr Kevorkian reached over to guide his hand.

Kevorkian straddled Tom's lap and began the search for a vein. His needle poked Tom in the shallow skin along the back of his left hand repeatedly, and Tom yelped in pain.

Dr Kevorkian stepped away. He turned off the video camera and returned to Tom. He tried the veins on the back of Tom's right hand and finally found one that would work. He restarted the video camera and began to prepare an intravenous line.

'Are you sure you want to go ahead now?' Dr Kevorkian asked.

Tom nodded again.

'We're ready to inject. We're going to inject in your right arm,' Dr Kevorkian said.

As he prepared to inject Seconal, a sedative, Tom Youk's body let out one final gasp. Thomas Youk's chin rested on his chest as the sedative flowed into his arm.

'Are you awake?' Dr Kevorkian asked.

Tom did not respond.

Dr Kevorkian injected a muscle relaxant, followed by potassium chloride, the drug that would stop Tom's heart quickly and pain-lessly. Tom's head tilted back. His mouth was open wide.

Kevorkian watched the electrocardiogram.

'Now there's a straight line,' Kevorkian pronounced. 'His heart has stopped.'

It took less than five minutes to end Tom Youk's life. Kevor-kian had done so less than three weeks after the enactment of a revised Michigan law making assisted suicide a felony punish-able by up to five years, and despite a court order banning him from assisting in suicide.

Dr Kevorkian left the house, and the Youks called a hospice worker to come and pronounce Tom deceased. The worker discovered a receipt for the package of medical records sent to Dr Kevorkian via Federal Express, which the family had left lying out. She called the police, and they immediately rushed to search the Youks' house.

Melody Youk notified Kevorkian of the events. He then contacted Mike Wallace of CBS's *60 Minutes* and arranged to have the tape shown – knowing that he would likely be charged with murder when the authorities saw the tape. It took some time for *60 Minutes* to edit the tape and schedule its airing. In the meantime, the Oakland county prosecutor was reluctant to charge Kevorkian for fear of losing the case, as others had before him. Kevorkian taunted the prosecutor publicly, but the prosecutor kept stalling.

Several weeks later, Jack called Ruth Holmes and asked to come and see her. Holmes was a trial consultant who specialised in determining the leanings of potential jurists by interpreting their handwriting. She forecast the psychological make-up of the five juries that had kept Dr Kevorkian out of jail, and became one of the few people he trusted. Ruth, expecting to have a cup of coffee and chat, had joked, 'OK, Jack, as long as you don't bring any bodies.'

Kevorkian didn't arrive until eleven that night. Ruth pulled out a midnight snack for him – his favourite white bread. Jack placed a plastic bag on the kitchen counter. Inside were a toothbrush and change of clothes. Jack told Ruth they were going to air the videotape he'd made of the Tom Youk medicide on *60 Minutes* that week.

'You know how the media will be,' he murmured, 'I can't go home.'

'Then stay here,' Ruth said.

On November 22nd, 1998, *60 Minutes* broadcast the videotape, which showed Dr Kevorkian giving the lethal injection to Thomas Youk. The programme triggered an intense debate within medical, legal and media circles. Kevorkian watched the broadcast from Ruth Holmes' living room with a group of friends. He was incredibly excited. He'd already formulated his plan of attack for the trial, and was eager to explain how he could win the case.

Three days later, the state of Michigan charged Jack Kevorkian with first-degree murder, violating the assisted suicide law and delivering a controlled substance without a licence. Prosecutors later dropped the suicide charge.

America saw the bombastic Dr Death on *60 Minutes*. When Mike Wallace asked Kevorkian what the difference was between murder and the service he had performed for Tom Youk, Kevorkian said, 'It could be manslaughter, not murder ... It's not necessarily murder, but it doesn't bother me what you call it. I know what it is. This could never be a crime in any society which deems itself enlightened.' He was intent on being prosecuted for his act, and so he didn't care what he said. He wanted a court case. He wanted to change the laws. But what America saw was a man who had caused another man to die, and who didn't seem bothered by what he'd done.

Mike Wallace asked, 'Did Tom know that you were making, in effect, an example [of him]?'

'Yes. And ... and I sensed some reluctance in him. I ... I did.'

'Because he had thought he was getting assisted suicide?'

'That's right. And ... and actually, this is better than assisted suicide. I explained that to him. It's better control. And then, he ... he did agree, which I ... I think ... I didn't force him to agree. He did agree. Maybe ...'

Once again, Jack wasn't being careful about what he was saying: Youk had initially asked for direct injection.

Wallace then asked, 'How do you know he agreed?'

'I had him sign, saying that he chose direct injection. And he ... and he signed this ... and he signed it.'

The interview gave even more ammunition for those that claimed that Dr Kevorkian was only involved with Tom Youk in order to gain publicity.

Mike Wallace announced, 'After more than 130 cases of assisted suicide, Dr Kevorkian says this is the first time that he taped the moment of death, and he says he did it to force his own arrest for euthanasia so he can have a trial to finally resolve whether he is right or the prosecutors are.'

Kevorkian replied, 'Either they go, or I go ... If-if I'm acquitted, they go because they know they'll never convict me. If I am convicted, I will starve to death in prison. So I will go. One of the two of us is going to go. And that's why I did this. The issue has got to be raised to the level where it is finally decided.'

'You were engaged in a political, medical, macabre publicity venture, right?'

'Probably.'

'And in watching these tapes, I get the feeling there's something almost ghoulish in your desire to see the deed done.'

'Well, that could be. I ... I can't argue with that. Maybe it is ghoulish. I don't know. It appears that way to you. I can't criticise you for that. But the main point is you … the last part of your statement, "that the deed be done".'

'[You] gave us the tape … to force their hand.'

'Absolutely, absolutely. I've got to force them to act. They must charge me, because if they do not, that means they don't think it's a crime. Because they don't need any more evidence, do they? Do you have to dust for fingerprints on this? … If you don't have liberty and self-determination, you got nothing. That's what this country is built on. And this is the ultimate self-determination: to determine when and how you're going to die when you're suffering.'

'And those who say that Jack Kevorkian — Dr Death — is a fanatic?'

'Zealot. No, not a tr— sure, you try to take a liberty away and I turn fanatic. That's what I'm fi— I'm fighting for me, Mike. Me. This is a right I want when I g— I'm 71. I'll be 71. You don't know what'll happen when you get older. I may end up terribly suffering. I want some colleague to be free to come and help me when I say the time has come. That's why I'm fighting, for me. Now that sounds selfish. And if it helps everybody else, so be it.'

During his stay with her, Ruth Holmes read him the letters he received and searched daily for positive articles that could encourage him. But Dr Kevorkian had a ruthless distaste for the slightest incompetence. She quietly bore his tirades and affronts. He derided her for the criticism he received in the press after the *60 Minutes* piece, but would then go out of his way to give press conferences in which he would ignore the suggested responses given him by legal council. She tolerated his outbursts as the price to pay for having such a noted doctor as a houseguest.

The Holmes family discovered that Jack didn't sleep much and didn't think others needed much sleep either. He would go to bed at one or two in the morning and wake up promptly at five, energetically tramping about the house. He coated the house in protective plastic pads, covering the edges of tables, chairs, the refrigerator and the stove, as he didn't want to accidentally bruise himself when roaming the house at night. Meals had to be carefully negotiated. They would catch him starting fires in the fireplace so that he could roast potatoes and marshmallows to go along with his toasted cheese sandwiches, and he wasn't happy until his food had a burnt carbon shell. He said burning food removed germs, but it was clear he also took pleasure in the charcoal taste.

When he stayed up late he initially only read or did jigsaw puzzles alone, but soon he grew accustomed to Ruth, her husband Peter and the occasional visits from daughter Sarah and son Nick. He hated seeing them watch TV, but when he discovered educational channels, he tried to get them to join him in watching a 'lovely' algebra programme on public television. Over time, the clatter of his morning routine diminished, and they often found him trying to 'quietly' play the piano rather than disturb them. Peter would come down early in the morning and banter with Jack over a cup of coffee, arguing politics, religion or economics. When visiting, Sarah was up next and they would play their flutes for an hour. Next Ruth would meet him for breakfast and they would go over letters he had received or legal issues he had to take into consideration. Jack would then retire to his room to paint. He gradually became a warm, flute-playing, Limerick-spinning grandfatherly figure they could count on for advice.

He often peeked out the curtains, looking for the telltale sign of snooping reporters, but it seemed like no one had discovered his hideout. One day a reporter banged on the front door. Kevorkian went into his room and drew the curtains and when Ruth finally opened the door, the reporter thrust a microphone in her face. She volunteered, 'I have no comment on Dr Kevorkian at this time. I will not address such issues from within my own home. There is a more appropriate time and place for any such inquiries.'

The reporter looked quizzically and responded, 'I just wanted your thoughts on the Monica Lewinsky scandal. What does her handwriting tell you about her? I'll ask about Kevorkian whenever he shows up in court. You don't happen to know where he is, do you?'

Ruth smiled guilelessly. 'He could be anywhere. He might be in one of your vans. Who knows, maybe he's hiding in my house.'

Geoffrey Fieger and Jack's other lawyers visited frequently to go over their strategy for the court case. If they were going to win, they had to convince the jury of Tom Youk's suffering and enable the jury to see Kevorkian the way Tom had – as the only person who could end his suffering.

Fieger warned Jack that the prosecutor would try and make him look like a monster. He also warned him not to repeat the finger-jabbing and screaming at the prosecutor that had gone on at the last trial. Kevorkian bristled, especially when Fieger told him he was trying to get the Youk videotape excluded as evidence. He didn't want the jury to see the tape; he knew that's what would get a conviction.

Kevorkian exploded. He wanted a conviction – he wanted to take his case to the Supreme Court. Fieger refused to help Kevorkian lose. To Feiger, having Jack acquitted of euthanasia in the county court would be groundbreaking in its own right, an important first step. Kevorkian's response was, 'Consider yourself fired.'

With no training in the law, nor any real idea as to courtroom procedure, he enlisted two young lawyers to replace Fieger and coach him on what to do. Neither had ever worked on a trial. One of the lawyers had even been fired from Fieger's law office, and it almost seemed as if that was exactly the reason Dr Kevorkian hired him. During the evenings spent with his new lawyers, Kevorkian's temper often got the better of him, and he would yell about their incompetence. He believed he knew what he was doing. He believed that he would get euthanasia acquitted in the Supreme Court. He talked of a Nobel Prize.

Kevorkian thought he had it all. He had a victim with a devastating terminal illness. The Youk family was supportive. The Oakland County prosecutor had been reluctant to bring charges for prior deaths. And Kevorkian had just been the 'star' of *Time*, the biggest news magazine in the world. But he had also rushed into the euthanasia of Tom Youk, sidestepping the one-month waiting period, ignoring the need for a psychological evaluation and, instead, trusting in his own judgment even though he barely knew Tom. He taped everything so that as far as the prosecution was concerned there was no doubt, no legal wrangling, as to who and what caused Tom Youk's death. Worst of all, he decided he knew enough of the law to represent himself in the biggest case of his life.

The case was a fiasco. Kevorkian made numerous factual errors regarding criminal law during his opening statement, and Circuit

Judge Jessica Cooper had to stop him and ask the jury to leave the room. She told him that he should consider getting legal representation. He refused. But this was certainly not the only legal abrogation that transpired.

The most monumental mistake, says Mayer Morganroth, Jack's present lawyer of account, was that one of Jack's young lawyers:

> ... contrary to the advisement from Jack and greater legal minds, [the lawyer] made the motion to dismiss the assisted suicide charge. Apparently his thought was that they would never convict Jack of murder. The motion was filed and they had a hearing in front of the judge. She was incredulous and asked if he was sure that was what he wanted to do ... She cautioned him that if he went ahead he couldn't put in any evidence for pain, suffering and the mental state of the deceased. This could only come in under assisted suicide. He still said yes so she denied his motion. The prosecution, hearing that, two weeks later dismissed the charge of assisted suicide.

This meant that Kevorkian's only defence was that the service he rendered should be legal. As she had stated, the judge did not allow any family members to testify as to Youk's wishes. Jack's lawyer argued that the jury should consider Youk's state of mind – that he wanted to die. But this was actually irrelevant. What was relevant was Jack's state of mind – that his intention was to not to kill Youk, but to end his suffering. This was not brought out in the trial because Jack was not allowed to have witnesses to attest to these truths. The prosecution was able to argue, without any witnesses and solely based on the tape, that Jack was an insensitive murderer.

★

The trial lasted just one-and-a-half days. (The OJ Simpson trial lasted nine-and-a-half months.) The jury found Dr Jack Kevorkian guilty. The Prosecuting Attorney recommended a sentence of five to seven years in a Federal Penitentiary; the judge sentenced him to 10 to 25 years in a maximum-security penitentiary in Michigan.

Jack Lessenberry, professor of Journalism at Wayne State University and a freelance journalist for the *New York Times*, the *Boston Globe*, the *Detroit Free Press, Vanity Fair* and numerous other publications, wrote in the *Oakland Press*:

> All the controversy surrounding his assisted suicides obscured some of his other achievements. Before Dr Jack Kevorkian there wasn't any pain management to speak of in America. The medical profession resisted giving painkillers in sufficient quantities to the terminally ill, fearing the patients could die or become addicted. Kevorkian, however, insisted that even if their lives could not be extended, they could at least live out their remaining weeks without torturous pain if they were given the proper amounts of pain medication. Medicide would be a last resort.
>
> Kevorkian trail-blazed physician assisted suicide in Oregon and Belgium through colleagues and patients. He prompted durable power of attorney, the ability to assign the right to make medical decisions to another person if you become incapacitated. He compelled advanced directives, statements about one's wishes should they become incapacitated: eg. 'DNR' – Do Not Resuscitate. Granted, he didn't work alone, but their acceptance and furtherance owe homage to Dr Jack Kevorkian.
>
> His fatal flaw emerged in his desire for the immortality bestowed upon many great human rights activists … The

self-destructive 'Dr Death' persona overwhelmed the eccentric, but kind aspects of his personality ... His normal self was quiet and rational ... But 'Dr Death' was all about flamboyance and emotion, about taking risks, about pushing people's buttons in order to get them into a fight ... Unfortunately ... the Kevorkian case became a launching pad to higher office for prosecutors intent on advancing their careers. His lawyers tried to take the case before the Supreme Court, but the court *refused to hear the* case. So, locked in a cell with another convicted murderer, Dr Jack Kevorkian has little chance of ever seeing the outside world again. He is known now only as Prisoner # 284797.

While in prison, Kevorkian's health began to fail. While walking through the 'recreation' yard he fell and broke two ribs. He suffered a double hernia and had to wait two years for corrective surgery. He is suffering from high blood pressure, cardiovascular disease, temporal arthritis, peripheral arthritis, adrenal insufficiency, chronic pulmonary obstruction disease and cataracts. His hepatitis C – contracted through research into blood transfusions – has reached dangerous levels.

In the most recent of his rare letters, he has told his friends that he is ready to die. He is at the end of his life, and there is little hope of him ever leaving prison. He is faced with the same situation Tom Youk was faced with, a terrifying future filled with misery. In his case, however, there is no one who can alleviate his suffering.

Chapter 2

GENOCIDE

It snowed in Pontiac, Michigan on May 26th, 1928, the day Jack Kevorkian was born. Satenig Kevorkian held her second child tight, smiling at the midwife, occasionally glancing at the white flecks of snow that floated outside her window. Levon Kevorkian stood on the small porch of their modest home and marvelled at the miracle. He had a home, a wife and finally a son who could continue the Kevorkian name.

Levon and Satenig were Armenian refugees who had narrowly escaped the butchery of the Turks during the dying days of the Ottoman Empire. Levon was born in the small village of Passen in northeast Turkey in 1891, while Satenig was born nine years later in the village of Govdun in central Turkey. If it hadn't been for the Turks, the two would never have met; a small consolation when compared to the holocaust perpetrated by the Turks on the Armenians in Asia Minor during World War I.

Armenia was then part of the Ottoman Empire – a dynastic state centred in what is now Turkey, founded in the late 13th century and dismantled after World War I. The Ottoman Empire had never been friendly to Armenians. The Armenians were

Christians, enduring for centuries in a land that had been a battleground for empires. In fact, Armenia was the first nation to adopt Christianity as its official state religion in 301 AD. For the Islamic rulers of the Ottoman Empire, however, they were nothing more than a blight in a holy land.

In the 19th century, the rest of the world began to notice the suffering of the Armenians. With the formation of the American Board of Commissioners for Foreign Missions in 1810, American Protestant missionaries began working in Asia Minor. Armenian language Bibles were distributed, and missionaries followed. When they discovered that the Ottoman Empire killed Muslims who showed an interest in Christianity, they turned their attention towards the Armenians, Assyrians and Greeks in the area. They considered the Armenian Apostolic Church 'backward', and so sought to save as many Armenians as possible by teaching them Protestant wisdom. An offshoot of this Protestant influence was an emphasis on the ideas of democracy, liberty and human dignity. Soon they had the Armenians believing that they had a right to freedom of expression and freedom from the oppression of the Ottoman Empire.

The push to assure the Armenians of basic rights inevitably led to war. Four Russo-Turkish wars raged through the 19th century. Although fought in part for control of the Balkans and Caucasus, the Russians made it quite clear they aimed to ease the suffering of Christians under Ottoman rule. Ironically, the efforts of the Protestant missionaries and Russian people to help their Christian brethren gave the sultan all the excuse he needed to begin his plan of extermination.

In 1894, a group of Armenians in the mountainous region of Sasoun defended themselves by force against abuses by the

Turks and Kurds. When news reached Sultan Abdul Hamid II he ordered his troops to quell the 'revolt'. The Ottoman troops raged through the region. They proceeded to corral the Armenian people, separating the men from the women. That night they raped the women, then bayoneted all the Armenians they could find. In the course of a few days, over 3,000 Armenians were dead.

Jack Kevorkian's parents were born in the midst of this violence. Their stories of how their families suffered while the rest of the world watched would foster the intense aversion to hypocrisy that motivated many of Jack's actions as an adult. Growing up, Kevorkian heard horrific tales of Armenian persecution. In the early part of the 20th century the Ottoman Empire implemented a systematic policy of rape and torture. The sultan released convicts from the prisons, armed them and sent them out with full permission to do as they would to the Armenians. The atrocities escalated. Jack heard stories of competitions between Turks who wanted to see who could commit the most heinous act. He was told thugs slaughtered entire villages, chopping the people into pieces that they threw into the wells and rivers until the very land seemed to bleed. Infants were cut from their mother's wombs. Children were raped, and left to wander the streets with horseshoes nailed to their feet. Many Armenians were crucified, the bloodthirsty throngs gathering around to laugh and point, yelling, 'Where is your Christ now?'

Though the rest of the world did little to stop the killings, some private aid agencies tried to save as many Armenian lives as possible. In 1912, Levon Kevorkian came across a group who were willing to smuggle him out of the country. He didn't want to leave his family behind, but he feared conscription into the slave labour battalions, where Armenian men were forced to build roads or used as human pack animals, and had already only narrowly escaped mobs that butchered his cousins and other relatives. He wouldn't have left if his father hadn't encouraged him: the family would be safe, his father assured him. The best way he could help was by earning enough money in some foreign land to pay for the escape of his brothers and sisters. So, with the assistance of missionaries, Levon eventually made his way to the Armenian community in Michigan and began work in an auto industry foundry. He saved his money, dreaming of the day when he could return to his country and save his family. But by 1915, his letters home were going unanswered.

The progressive 'Young Turks' had taken over from the Sultan in 1908, but nationalists took over in the group and by 1915 the Armenian Genocide was at full force. Two million Armenians living in Turkey were ousted from their historic homeland through forced deportation and massacre. Levon would discover in the aftermath of World War I that the Turks slaughtered at least 800,000 Armenians in 1915 alone – and he was the only Kevorkian to have survived the slaughter.

Although Satenig Kevorkian often turned silent when Jack and his two sisters asked about her life during the holocaust, they learned a few telling details of her ordeal. She came from a relatively wealthy family and they were protected from the atrocities for some time by her father's influence. But her father miscalculated. He thought the situation would improve when the Young Turks took power and when the violence began again, he assumed that Europe would swiftly intervene. By the time he realised his folly it was too late. The Turks executed him along with other intellectuals, and after his death, Satenig's family was forced into the 1915 death march. As World War I raged, the Turkish government decided upon the systematic extermination and forced deportation of most of the Armenian population. The deportation became a death march, with extreme violence and deprivation leading to the death of an estimated 600,000 marchers. Satenig's entire village – along with 1.75 million other Armenians – were uprooted and forced to walk for months and hundreds of miles until they reached the hot desert sands of Syria and Mesopotamia. Satenig saw her younger brother killed before her eyes. Her mother fell ill and died during the trek. Her younger sister, who had been considered the most beautiful girl in the village, was raped and brutalised throughout the march – she finally died of cholera. Arabs took another of her sisters into a harem. Satenig would later discover that she eventually escaped and settled in Lebanon.

Satenig managed to escape from the death march. Surviving on whatever scraps of food she could find, she continued alone until she finally reached Basra, where a ship took her to Marseilles. She eventually encountered some relatives in Paris who were able to connect her with her brother Peter, who had emigrated to Argentina before the war. It was Peter who brought her to Pontiac, Michigan, where they both tried to begin a new life.

In Pontiac, the Armenians who had survived the Turkish massacre clung tightly together. Since many Armenian survivors were the only ones in their family to escape death, they protected others in the community and assisted the Armenian immigrants flooding into the country. They found comfort in the church and in the company of the other refugees. With each other, they could talk about the horrific images that crowded their nightmares.

It was through the Armenian community that Levon and

Satenig first met. They walked the peaceful streets of Pontiac together, marvelling at the calm of this new country in which they found themselves. Satenig was not ready for any kind of romantic relationship; the scars of her ordeal were too fresh. It helped that Levon was not interested in one either. With Satenig it was as if he was speaking to a younger sister again, and so he coached her on the dangers of this new land, the rituals and rhythms of American society. Working in America before she had even dreamed of the possibility of escape, he was streetwise in a way that she would never be. In turn, Satenig had been fortunate enough to attend school for a number of years in Armenia, and was one of the most literate of the Armenian immigrants in the area. She helped him as he wrote letters and attempted to find out what happened to his family, and together they took on the challenge of learning the English language. Their friendship became a love that could heal old wounds. Together they felt like family, and so they decided to marry and create a new family to replace the ones that the Ottoman Empire had ripped from them.

It was clear that though the rest of the world felt that what had happened to the Armenians was a tragedy, nobody was all that interested in putting an end to the violence or in helping the Armenians mend their shattered lives. As World War I ended, Europe finally began to consider punishing the Central Powers for war crimes and atrocities. Woodrow Wilson announced his ambitious Fourteen Points, emphasising self-determination and justice for Armenians and other oppressed people. But as Levon and Satenig watched in disbelief, the world again shirked its responsibilities. The young couple could scarcely believe it when the headlines in the local newspaper announced that the US delegation had voted against the War Crimes Commission.

Republican isolationists succeeded in mobilising opposition to Wilson's plan, and other world leaders, fearful of antagonising the Turks and losing access to the rich oil fields of the Middle East, soon abandoned the quest for retribution.

Although photographic evidence of the atrocities in Armenia had reached the West, and despite the overwhelming volume of eyewitness testimony, US officials retreated from their previous condemnation of the Ottoman Empire. The oil wealth of the Middle East was up for grabs, and World War I had taught the US that it needed oil if it was to be a major player on the world stage. Rather than offend their new friends by reminding them of the atrocities they had committed, US officials began to re-imagine what had happened.

As the world slowly turned away from the Armenian survivors and ignored the tragedy, Levon and Satenig Kevorkian felt an increasing sense of betrayal. They taught their son that politicians and government were not concerned about the truth, the outside world was full of deception and people could only trust their own family. It was a principle that would guide Jack throughout his life – there were very few figures of authority who earned and kept his trust.

Chapter 3

THE RISE OF A REBEL

Satenig wanted to name her son Murad, after a famous and courageous Armenian guerrilla fighter who fought valiantly to protect his people. She wanted her son to have the same courage as his namesake. Levon, however, wanted to call his young son Jacob. It was a solid, respectable name, one that would fit in well in America. With that name, the boy would blend in at school and people would think of him as an American instead of as the son of immigrants. Satenig also wanted her son to have every advantage, so if her husband said that the right name made that possible, then she was willing to go along. At home, though, she continued to call her young son Murad. The world would know him as Jacob, the patriarch of the 12 tribes of Israel, but inside, her son would forever be Murad, a brave soldier who was willing to sacrifice his life for what was right.

The doctor who signed the birth certificate wasn't all that concerned with what the boy was named. Whether he had difficulty understanding the Kevorkians' accented pronunciation, or because he was too busy to care, he nevertheless illegibly scrawled a name on the birth certificate. That illegible name was later interpreted by a teacher as Jack, so Jack he became. It was a nice Christian name and an acceptable shortening of his given name Jacob. In time, Levon gave him the nickname 'Joe' and this became his only name with the neighbourhood kids. Whichever name he was called by, throughout his life Jack Kevorkian made an impression few who met him could forget.

The Kevorkian neighbourhood was a far cry from the chaos of Armenia. The family lived on a side street just a short distance from downtown Pontiac. The family houses and duplexes were (and still are) close together, with 'postage-stamp' size front lawns. Although not wealthy, Jack's father was able to purchase three lots and built the house and garage himself.

Perhaps because the Great Depression left many houses vacant and made the area more affordable, a variety of working-class immigrants settled in the area. Greeks, Italians and Germans lived in harmony with Mexicans, Filipinos and African Americans. Though racial tensions could have been an issue, age alone seemed to be the only divider between gangs of playmates. In Jack's group, the boys sometimes pummelled each other to establish who was top dog, but all the kids had immigrant parents, and nobody seemed to care which country you'd come from.

The boys played marbles and kick-the-can during the day and a spooky night-time hide-and-seek. If the streets weren't too busy they played touch football, and baseball in the open fields. When bored, they joined the girls playing hopscotch and jump rope. Every spring the air was filled with kites, and Jack would fly his own creation, which he'd frugally craft out of string, newspapers and starch paste. In winter the kids turned anything flat into a sled, then competed for speed or distance on the slick, frozen surfaces of the paved streets. Jack loved bicycling and would often venture as far as the woods of Walled Lake, 20 miles away. They were outdoor kids stuck in a city, and only ambled home after hearing their names yelled a few times by their exasperated mothers. Of course, on the rare occasion that their fathers called for them they ran home immediately.

Levon worked hard to provide a stable home and to keep his family clothed and fed during the Depression. He made sure his daughters Margaret (Margo), two years older than Jack, and Flora, one-and-half-years younger, went to school and encouraged them to do the best they could, but his attention was focused on Jack. Jack was his only son, the only one who could carry the Kevorkian name. Levon felt it was his responsibility to make sure that his son made the right decisions. When he talked with the boy, he emphasised that he should always do what was right, help when he could, and obey authority.

According to both Jack and Flora, their parents were strict, 'old-worldish' and introspective. They took great pride in their children – especially Jack. In her later years, Flora would often speak of her parents' preference for Jack, explaining repeatedly (perhaps with just a hint of resentment) that 'he was brilliant, just brilliant'.

Jack was also the boy the other kids wanted to follow. He would lead them into the abandoned houses in the neighbour-hood and command them to strip them of any usable piece of wood. They would then use the wood to make swords and shields for games of fencing. They used the leftover wood to fuel small pit fires in vacant lots and roasted the few potatoes their mothers could spare. It was where Jack began to develop his eccentric taste in food – he became addicted to the taste of the hot, soft, white potatoes covered by thin peels of charcoal. In the stripped houses the boys ran on wood beams and swung on joists in games of tag that occasionally left them bruised, but they learned not to show that they were hurt.

One time Jack fell and fractured his right arm. His arm dangled at his side, numb, but when he moved even the slightest bit, pain would wrench his body. At the hospital the doctor had to reset the overlapping fracture more than once, finally using a metal support to keep the arm in a wing-like position for several weeks. Through it all, Jack didn't cry. For the boys, that was all the evidence of manliness they needed to see. Jack was a leader to be followed.

Unfortunately for Levon, the first authority Jack was to battle against was his father. Levon was appalled when, in the 1930s, he heard rumours of impending war, but Jack was excited by the prospect. He recruited an army of neighbourhood kids, and marched and drilled them everywhere. He designed their rifles, including bayonets, which they meticulously cut and shaped with saw and files. They also had a howitzer constructed from a log and bicycle wheels. Jack made papier-mâché German and doughboy helmets using washbowls as forms. General Jack Kevorkian, aka Blackjack Pershing, also designed and made medals from cardboard that were replicas of World War I awards and only the truly brave were bestowed with this honour. The boys used wooden 'potato mashers' in lieu of hand grenades. Thrown within ten feet of an 'enemy soldier' he was 'dead', or supposed to be, as arguments were frequent and loud.

They held their war games in the vacant acreage across from St Joseph's Hospital in Pontiac. Heavily treed hills rolled away from a broken down brick building, creating a perfect battlefield and bunker for their war games. The boys had lunches made for all-day episodes. Jack designated the areas: the Belleau Woods, Somme, Verdun and Vimy Ridge. The rest of the boys barely knew where Detroit was, let alone the World War I battlefields of France and Belgium, but Jack's imagination made the whole world available to them.

Although the patriotic fervour of the times inspired many boys to play war games, Levon had expected his boy to be different. He had stressed at home how he detested war, where young men were always being sent off to die in battlefields over imaginary boundaries, but where nothing ever seemed to change or be accomplished. The world leaders would meet at the end of their wars and declare that good had prevailed, and then economic trade would resume and apologies given and accepted by their erstwhile enemy. A few years later, more fighting would break out. The vicious circle of war and peace fed on the lives of young men, and the suffering of the innocents hidden behind battle lines continued through it all. But Jack felt that soldiers could bring justice and peace, and he felt that he had to side with the Americans because they were fighting on the side of good. Levon tried to argue with his son, but Jack, like Levon himself, wasn't one to change his mind easily. Levon hoped that Jack would outgrow his naïveté before the war machine destroyed him for it.

When Levon and Satenig told their son about their ordeals in Armenia, they stressed that it was only by God's grace that they survived. They repeated the common understanding held in the local Armenian Apostolic church that their suffering in Armenia had been redemptive, that it was better to live their lives with compassion and dignity than to dwell on past wrongs and desire revenge. One simply had to accept what God had allotted, and strive to be a good Christian in dealing with the repercussions of tragedy. This philosophy didn't make any sense to Jack. In the church they talked of justice and redemption, but the Armenian holocaust defied those words. The Turks had slaughtered his people without retribution. The survivors had nightmares, but the perpetrators denied it ever happened. It seemed to him that the words 'justice' and 'redemption' were just words used to disguise moments in mankind that were pure evil. If such terrible things occurred, didn't it at least bring up the possibility that God didn't care, or, maybe, that God didn't exist at all? If God's son could walk on water, something that seemed scientifically impossible to Jack, couldn't he stop genocide? He repeatedly raised the conundrum in Sunday school until he was 12 or 13, and when no one could give a satisfactory explanation he stopped going, much to his parents' chagrin.

But Levon was to win the battle about Jack's education. Jack loved baseball. While other boys were just beginning to learn the rules of the game, Jack was busy memorising statistics. He began to put on a daily show for the neighbourhood kids, calling a play-by-play as he threw a tennis ball against the front steps of his house. Depending on how the ball hit the steps, he called either a single, double, triple or homerun, imitating the voice of Jack Graney, the announcer for his favourite team, the Cleveland Indians.

'With that triple, Earl Averill is batting a blistering .322,' he'd say, and the kids would edge closer, cheering as if they were hearing a live game on the radio. Jack became their eyes and ears into a baseball world that existed only in the twists of his imagination. For Jack, it created a place all his own, far away from his parents' nightly remembrances of loved ones lost in distant Armenia.

Jack often thought about how he could channel his talent. If he worked hard at it, he might be able to go to Cleveland and train under Jack Graney himself. He knew he would be great because it was what he loved to do. He knew he had talent, and in America a kid with talent could go far – or so it was portrayed in all the books and movies. His friends said he turned baseball into poetry. But for Levon, Jack's ambition made little sense. How could anyone make a living talking about a game? What fools would ever support a man pursuing something so trivial? It was all right for children to daydream about fame and fortune, but when they started to believe in their own daydreams, it was time for a good parent to step in and bring them back to earth. Jack was smart, that was clearly evident, but Levon felt it was his duty to steer his son towards college and the possibility of a job where you wore a tie and ordered men like Levon around.

Margo and Flora were also gifted children, but Satenig and Levon didn't put as much pressure on them as they did Jack. They wanted their daughters to succeed but, as was common at the time, their standard for girls was lower than what was expected from boys. A girl, if she was smart and worked hard, could become a secretary or a teacher; appropriate jobs for women. The best thing a woman could do was to use her intelligence as bait to lure a good man into marriage.

So while Jack was expected to work hard in school and climb the education ladder, Margo and Flora were taught the skills that Levon and Satenig felt best ornamented a woman's beauty: music and art. Both sisters were gifted with beautiful soprano voices, but neither they nor their parents considered the possibility of a career in music. Flora, the youngest, showed an artistic bent, so her parents provided her with paint and drawing materials. For

Margo, Levon found a used upright piano with keys so mottled it looked like a gapped-tooth six-year-old. They couldn't afford a piano instructor, but it turned out that Margo didn't really need one. She had the ability to play by ear, and would entertain her family by playing back popular songs she'd heard only a few times. To improve her music expertise she taught herself how to read musical scores. Jack's lifelong love of Bach had its conception from hearing Margo play Bach's French Suites.

Jack resented the fact that activities considered acceptable for his sisters were considered frivolous for him. He loved drawing and painting, and tried to soak up as much knowledge as he could by watching Flora work. He listened intently when Margo sat down at the piano and made mental notes that he hoped he could put to use after he finished his education. To his frustration, the only thing his parents seemed to care about, though, was how well he did in school. Even his sisters argued that his education was far more important than art or music. The Kevorkian family expected greatness of him, and it was as if they all made an agreement to work together to keep him from getting sucked into fantasies of a life in sports or the arts.

Jack and his sisters had their petty squabbles, but it always seemed as if the girls retreated from their arguments. They would eventually help or defend him, always doing more for him than he did in return and, like Levon, making sacrifices to give Jack a chance at a better life.

Jack didn't want the sacrifices. He was being spoiled because he was the brilliant heir apparent. Though he enjoyed the attention from his family, he recognised that his sisters weren't getting the same opportunities. Margo was at the top of her class, and Flora too was obviously brilliant. All the Kevorkian kids ended up winning first place in the citywide spelling bees, even though none of them studied for the event. It was clear to Jack that his sisters could achieve as much, if not more, than he, if only given the chance. Levon, however, wouldn't hear of it. Jack may have been a smart kid, but Levon wasn't about to take parenting suggestions from his son.

Jack loved his dad, but he felt Levon didn't understand him or keep up with modern times. Levon was filled with all the old-fashioned ideas of Armenia, and was satisfied with his working-class status; he was used to taking orders. Even in America, Levon still acted as if trouble was just around the corner. Due in part to the language barrier, Levon always felt as if he was an outsider, and he expected some American official to come any day and tell him he had to leave. He was unfailingly polite to whoever he met — it was wise to be courteous, Levon felt, since he was clearly a guest in America.

It would take years for Jack to fully appreciate his father, and as a child he viewed his father's advice more as an annoyance than good counsel. His father had lost his job at a foundry at the start of the Great Depression and consequently started his own excavation company. Pulling together a band of Armenians who knew how to do the work, Levon built a solid business that his family could rely on. Though he was an opinionated man, whose bad temper occasionally got the better of him, he was honest and hard working, and asked for nothing else from his working crews. Word of his honesty and diligence soon spread about the Pontiac area and he was rewarded with continued contracts. But all Jack could see was how his dad would lower his eyes and subjugate himself to the men who hired him, how he listened to their every word out of fear that one misstep would lead to him losing the job.

Levon appreciated his son's intelligence, even casual bystanders would remark on it when they overheard the boy speaking. From an early age his son read everything and anything he could get his hands on: books at the library, magazines at the barbershop, even stray pages from newspapers that the bushes in front of their house snagged on windy days. Anything the boy read, he remembered, wielding facts and figures in arguments as if his life depended on winning the debate. Levon knew it wasn't likely that generous teachers would surround his son throughout his life and keep him motivated, so he tried to instil a work ethic that would last the boy's life.

Jack couldn't understand the silly rules people wanted him to observe, arbitrary decisions made to mould him into what they thought he should become. Church, school and family all wanted to dictate his life, but he was never willing to compromise. In confrontation, diplomats might soften their voice, adjust their tone to make their point more acceptable, but Jack, never the diplomat, lashed out with gusto. In school, the teachers became his targets, and as he took them on the kids admired and even adulated him.

Even so, Jack never felt like he completely fitted in with the crowd. He was smarter than they were; and his intellect created an invisible barrier. He couldn't connect with either the kids or most of the teachers, mainly because more often than not they couldn't grasp the complexity of the subject matters in which he was interested. He tried to bridge the gap with humour. He would clown around in class, humiliating the teacher in arguments usually laced with jokes. His defiance was intended to amuse his audience, but it only further isolated him, as if he were an actor performing a role before a paying crowd. Some of these kids later echoed this, describing Jack as 'brilliant', 'athletic' and 'comical', but also 'distant'.

While the other kids struggled through their lessons at their desks, Jack would quickly finish and poke fun at the teachers with cartoons he drew in his notebook. On one occasion when he was asked to write on the blackboard, he took a piece of chalk in both hands, wrote the answer with his right hand, and simultaneously wrote the mirror image with his left. On another occasion, in middle school, while the teacher was talking about the Panama Canal Jack went to the blackboard and drew a mural of the canal full of ships, surrounded by mountains, palm trees, tropical birds and mules hauling drays. Schoolmates recall watching in amazement as this beautiful vista materialised from ordinary coloured chalk.

The kids thought of him as a rebel and a joker, but they also recognised his brilliance. Even the teachers knew they couldn't fully engage his intellect, and they tried to get him to be more patient with the other students who had to labour over the same material. In the end, most teachers just tried to keep him busy as a way to keep him quiet.

When he was nine years old, his 5th grade teacher tried to restrain Jack's exuberance by making him captain of the safety patrol. Initially, Jack didn't want the honour, but when he realised the position came with a uniform he changed his mind. The uniform made him stand out, made him feel as if the entire school was recognising his importance. He took pride in the ornate belt that came with the position, and welcomed rainy days because he could swagger from corner to corner in his special waterproof cape, monitoring patrol stations with his lieutenants.

But being captain of the safety patrol didn't keep Jack out of trouble for long. Early in his 6th grade year, after having finished his

assigned lessons, Jack decided to amuse himself by shooting spit-
balls (small pieces of paper wadded up and chewed to wet them)
with a rubber band at the classroom clock. The other kids began
to notice the spitball-covered clock, and soon the entire class had
stopped work to point at the clock and laugh. The teacher yelled
at the kids to get back to work, but her voice was drowned out by
the laughter. To Jack's surprise, she stared at him, her eyes welling
up with tears. She put her head in her hands and cried. When the
class finally quieted down, and she had regained some of her composure, she glared at Jack and walked out of the classroom. A friend
turned to Jack and said, 'Boy, you're gonna get it now!' Jack wasn't
concerned about punishment. It was expected. What bothered him
most was that he'd made his teacher cry. He didn't know how to
apologise for that.

After half an hour the teacher returned and asked him to gather
his books and proceed to the principal's office. Jack geared himself
for the worst. The principal, Ms Cleveland, was a stern 60-year-
old who had previously warned him that the next time he walked
into her office would be his last. Jack expected a moralistic ser-
mon and some minor punishment. Instead, Ms Cleveland told
him to take his books and go home – and not to come back until
he brought his father with him.

Jack was terrified. Teachers and principals didn't frighten him.
The worst they ever did was to scold him or give him detention.
But involving his father was another matter altogether. He just
didn't want to think of how his father would react.

When Margo came home from school Jack told her everything. He told her how sorry he was, that he'd been bored and
hadn't meant to make the teacher cry. He pleaded with her to
help. Maybe she could talk to Levon and fix the situation for him.

She had a better idea, which may have been the beginning of a lifelong pattern of Margo being Jack's confidant, organiser and troubleshooter.

The next day Margo went to school with Jack. She explained to Ms Cleveland that Levon and Satenig had to go to work (which was a lie – Satenig did not work), but that they had sent her to deal with the situation. She told the principal that Jack had promised that he would not repeat his misbehaviour, and that his parents were intent on holding him to his word.

Jack vowed that he would accept whatever punishment she had in store. Ms. Cleveland smiled, and told him that she was not letting him go back to his 6th grade class. Instead, he was to report the next day to Eastern Junior High School.

The promotion worked well for Jack. Now he had a new set of classes to study for and a different band of boys to win over. The challenge kept him occupied for a while and quieted his rebelliousness. As an added bonus, Levon was proud of him. As far as his father knew the promotion was based on academic excellence.

Jack was proud that his academic achievements pleased his parents. At least in school he could be what they expected of him. And as his artistic flair turned towards mechanical drawings in junior high, he began to tell Levon that he was interested in becoming a civil engineer. The smile on his father's face was worth more to him than all of the years of straight As in school.

But Jack wouldn't be Jack if he had left it at that. Soon he was playing the clown in junior high and disrupting classes again. He was popular with the other kids, and in 8th grade they chose him to be on the student council. In order to be on the student council, however, a student needed not only good grades in academic subjects, but also good marks for personal behaviour. Within a few weeks Jack was kicked off the student council. Jack would later say that the ejection didn't bother him, that he didn't care for picayune junior high politics, that he didn't want to be like the cookie cutter students on the council, destined to become religious Republicans. But still, the rejection hurt.

It didn't help that boys and girls in junior high were making their first forays into courtship. Being the youngest in his class, Jack felt completely out of place. He could talk to a girl, but he didn't know how to tell them he liked them. Skinny, bookish and very young, he felt as if the girls didn't even notice him. He tried to engage them in intellectual conversation because, after all, wasn't the mind the true measure of a person? But the girls only giggled and scurried away. He was funny and intelligent, but he didn't seem to be anybody's idea of a boyfriend.

Levon seemed to sense the sadness in his son. One day he returned from work with a stray white poodle he had found on the jobsite. He gave the dog to Jack, knowing that Jack would have an obedient and faithful friend in the dog, and also hoping that taking care of it would teach Jack responsibility. Jack named the dog 'Wooly' and the two became inseparable. Jack took Wooly with him wherever he could, and spent hours just playing with and petting him. After school, Jack would race home on his bike, eager to meet up with the bouncing little white ball of a dog that yapped at him with love. Then one day Jack raced home only to find Wooly's broken body by the side of the road. He took his friend into the backyard and laid him on the grass, crying uncontrollably. It was his first experience with the death of a friend, but more than that, it felt as if it was the death of love itself. He had opened himself up and been loved in return, and now with this loss the pain was almost unbearable. He vowed he would never let it happen again. This minor incident made a big impression on Jack (he talked about it often), and may have impacted his relationships in later life.

By the time Jack entered high school aged 15 he had given up on the idea of having a girlfriend. Romance was an unnecessary diversion, he felt, and it was far more important for him to cultivate his mind. He believed the girls weren't interested in him anyway, so he didn't consider it much of a sacrifice. On his best days, he simply considered it a postponement of love. Some day, after he had achieved his success, he might find an intellectual equal, and they could form a family without too much of the awkwardness of small talk and dating. On his worst days, he envisioned a lifetime alone, as if he had taken a vow of celibacy and solitude in order to join the priesthood of knowledge.

Jack thought that being a cartoonist for the *Pontiac Tomahawk*, the high school monthly magazine, might be a safe outlet for the humour. That, however, didn't last long. The students enjoyed Jack's barbs at the school, the teachers and even local politicians. When he decided to make fun of Thanksgiving, drawing a caricature of the principal as the turkey, the school administration saw to it that he was kicked off the magazine. Most of the students felt that the punishment was too severe, and Jack enjoyed a bit of popularity as a result. Once again, the students elected him to the student council, almost as if to say they were sorry for what had happened to him with the magazine – but once again his low marks for social behaviour ended a short stint.

Every effort at connecting with the students or teachers seemed to run into an administrative roadblock. If he tried humour, a teacher would yell at him because his behaviour was inappropriate.

46

But when he tried to talk to instructors about the exciting things he was reading and learning on his own, he was greeted by blank stares. The teachers couldn't understand him, so when he tried to engage them in intellectual conversation, they stared at him coldly as if he had just made another inappropriate joke. The hip crowd in the school enjoyed Jack's sense of humour, but many of them viewed him as an eccentric bookworm. It wasn't normal for a person to read so much and work so hard in school. They couldn't pronounce half the words he used when he was making his philosophical arguments, let alone understand them. He just wasn't like the other kids.

Jack retreated within himself. He still tried to mix with his schoolmates, but he now began to focus more on what he considered important. If others liked him, fine. If not, he convinced himself he wouldn't care. He began to undertake projects at home and, enlisting the aid of a few of the neighbourhood kids who still liked to tag around with him, he constructed a chemical lab in the basement of his house. His friends were fascinated. He built a vacuum tube radio and showed his friends how to make their own. Childhood friend Vanig Godoshian later said he spent a career in electronics because of Jack's early radio days. He showed them how to make gunpowder. He helped them make small packets of potassium nitrate that they could scatter on the sidewalks – anyone who stepped on one would receive a surprising jolt. He even made a fire extinguisher to protect the household. He knew he wouldn't make any mistakes in his lab, but just in case, it would be better to have something on hand than have to deal with Levon if he came home to find the house had burned down.

Jack also soon discovered that the best way to satisfy his intellectual curiosity was to expose himself to books written in other languages. If he could read and write in other languages, he could feel a part of the intellectual discoveries going on in other parts of the world. Unfortunately, because of World War II, only Spanish was being taught in school. Even the Latin class had been discontinued. Jack joined the Spanish class, but soon began to study German and Japanese on his own, poring over any book he could find in the library. Since the country was at war, he felt it prudent to know the language of the enemy. In a few months he was fluent in both German and Japanese and planned on joining the intelligence corps as soon as he was old enough to volunteer. He tried to teach his friends basic words and phrases to make their war games more realistic, but soon gave up on the effort. The reward for teaching his friends a few words was far less rewarding than the intellectual satisfaction he gained from spending the same amount of time trying to decipher books in their native languages.

Levon brought Jack to work for him in the summers. He told Jack he wanted to show him how disciplined a man needed to be in order to succeed. But, secretly, he also hoped having his son watch him at work would motivate the boy to strive for a white-collar life. In fact, while thoroughly enjoying the work, Jack promised himself he would never make it his career. He would never become one of the invisible men that laid sewer pipe throughout Pontiac.

Jack arrived late for graduation and decided to stand behind the last rows and observe the proceedings. A classmate noticed him, grabbed him by the arm, and told him he should be sitting up front. Jack protested that he was comfortable where he was, until the friend informed him that, as one of the top 10 per cent of the class he was supposed to sit in the first row.

It was a pleasant shock for Jack. He had no idea that the school handed out such honours or that his grades merited any special recognition. All the detentions and demerits for bad behaviour meant nothing now. Intelligence had won out, and he hadn't needed to be a docile, slavish conformist in order to survive high school.

That night Jack entertained his friends and family by playing a mean boogie-woogie on the piano. He had gone through high school his own way, dealt with all the humourless, slow-witted teachers, and emerged victorious. And now he was going to college, to the prestigious University of Michigan College of Engineering. Levon and Satenig stood proudly behind their son, smiling as his fingers flew across the piano keys. Their dreams of greatness for Jack were coming true. He was the kind of man who could create his own destiny.

Chapter 4

THE FORMATIVE YEARS

Jack worked alongside his father again in the summer of 1945. He may have preferred to hide from the torrid heat in the cool confines of a library, but respect for his father outweighed his preference. As long as he lived at home during the summer, Jack was expected to work. And Jack actually thrived on the hard, physical labour. He loved working alongside his dad.

Levon enjoyed the look on the city engineers' faces when he told them his scrawny son was going to be an engineer. It surprised them when Levon said that the young man struggling with a pick and shovel intended to be their equal. Jack wasn't going to be a common labourer, Levon liked to tell them. Jack had intelligence. Jack was going to be their boss some day. When his father said these things, Jack just stared at the ground. He liked the praise, it made him feel good to know that his accomplishments made his dad proud, but he felt like little more than a trophy carted out to the work site. Just the same, Jack enrolled in civil engineering at the University of Michigan in Ann Arbor.

If Jack was going to create an exciting career for himself, he was going to have to work hard. He couldn't afford to be a child any more. He would have to make sure he outworked everyone around him, because if he failed in achieving his own path, the only alternative was to lay pipe alongside his father and dream about what could have been. So when the newspapers announced VJ Day on August 15th, 1945, Jack ended his childhood. He gathered up the squadron of homemade model Japanese fighter planes and hung them in a tree. One by one, he set them on fire. He promised himself he would never waste time with childish games again.

While other freshmen busily scouted out the local night-time hotspots, Jack toured the campus, jotting notes on library and building closing times. As others sat down over a beer and indulged themselves, Jack surrounded himself with books – philosophy, history and music, it didn't matter. The college library had more books than he could ever possibly hope to read, but he promised himself that he would make a significant dent in the stacks. He made the library a second home. Sometimes when he saw the other students ambling about, babbling inanely about beer and women, he yearned to be a part of such simple friendships. If a student approached him, Jack was friendly enough, prone to show off the cartoons he scribbled in the margins of his notebooks, or to recite the latest string of Limericks that had come to mind while he was in the shower. But the choice, to him, seemed clear. He could be like the other students, divvying his energies between the social and intellectual worlds, obediently accepting the life and career track that his course schedule put him on, or he could fill his mind with so much knowledge that the path of his life would forever be his to choose.

Despite his dedication, his first semester did not go as well as expected. In high school Jack was a straight 'A' student and top of his class – at University of Michigan he did not get straight As; in fact, he was in middle of all his classes academically. One of the requirements for his civil engineering major was analytical geometry. Angle measurements, proofs and slide rules were easy enough to master, but he was bored. He was expected to look at diagrams of triangles and rhombuses and care about whether or not he could calculate the length of a side. Geometry seemed irrelevant, and the homework even more so. The problem sets he was given didn't vary much from day to day. There again was the same triangle, the same trapezoid. The questions were slightly different, but the same formulas, theorems and proofs came into play. He felt like little more than a machine clicking through a tried and true system of logical deduction. It was a waste of his abilities, and he resented the repetitive drudgery.

His foreign language courses were far more interesting. Though the US Army Japanese language school was but a remnant of its wartime size, two instructors still took on intermediate level students. When the instructors found out that Jack was a freshman, they told him there was no way he could join the class. Only the best students from the previous year's beginning Japanese class were eligible. Jack thought he was too advanced for a beginner's class, so he pleaded his case in Japanese.

The instructors stared at him and asked where he had learned to speak so well. Jack grinned and told them he'd learned from books. They asked how he learned the proper pronunciation. Jack again said from a book – one that showed how to phonetically pronounce the words. He'd read that one over a dozen times. The instructors wondered if he could read and write Japanese characters. 'Not yet,' he said, 'but maybe next week.'

The instructors laughed and told Jack that he'd be completely lost in the class and would never be able to catch up. Jack vowed to prove them wrong, and stormed off to the library.

The class was a small one, with only three other students. They were shocked when Jack, a freshman, first walked in. When the instructor told them that Jack planned on catching up to their level, the students thought he was joking.

Jack blundered his way through the first class. The other students sighed in frustration; he was going to slow them down. The instructors openly laughed at Jack's mistakes, eager to humble the arrogant kid who thought he could jump right into their intermediate class.

Jack quickly developed a battle strategy. When he wasn't in class he was in the library studying. Outside of the time necessary to keep up with his other classes, he devoted every waking moment to deciphering the Japanese script. He kept himself going by drinking a dozen cups of coffee a day, and every few hours he used a donut as an energy boost. When Jack began to dream in Japanese, he knew he was getting somewhere. Within a month, he was the best student in the class.

Jack found that German was an easier language to learn, so he enrolled in German I and II in the same semester to save time. Other students had to pause to mentally translate foreign words into English, then translate their answer back into the other language. For Jack, it was as if he could throw a switch in his mind. One moment he would be thinking in English, the next, in German or Japanese or Armenian, whatever the situation required. One instructor suggested that Jack consider a career in translation. It was high praise, but Jack didn't give the suggestion much thought. A translator was nothing more than a bridge between languages, a tool other people used. Being a translator seemed as boring as a civil engineer trapped into drafting designs for inconsequential projects.

After some soul searching he decided he didn't really want to be an engineer, but wasn't sure what he wanted to do. In the interim, he decided to enroll in the so-called softer sciences, botany and biology.

After three semesters in college, he had racked up 57 credit hours, and when an instructor informed him that medical school required only a total of 90 credit hours, he seriously began to set his sights on becoming a doctor. Doctors were in great demand, so a career in medicine would always keep him employed. Medicine was also an escalating branch of learning; great advancements were being made every day, and he could see himself becoming a part of the medical revolution. As a doctor, he could conduct research, make a good income and enjoy the respect of others. Medicine would be perfect for him.

There was of course the issue of his father. When Jack returned home and told his parents that he wished to drop engineering his father was extremely disappointed, but this turned to admiration and pride when Jack explained that he wished to be a medical doctor. For his parents, all that mattered was that Jack use his intellect to find a respectable life. Jack, however, wanted more.

It struck him one day in the library that mankind advanced by recording the discoveries of others and then exploring deeper. The challenge as a human being was to find the way in which one could further that exploration. Jack was confident that the best way for him to do that was by exploring the science of life itself. He was sure that if he focused, he would find a way to do something important.

Jack launched himself into the next semester with renewed vigour. He loaded up on biology and botany courses. He camped out in the student centre cafeteria most days, frantically jotting notes as he tore through his books. The cafeteria seemed like the perfect place for him. Whenever he began to feel tired, he could get up and grab another donut or cup of coffee to refuel. With his table coated with papers and donut crumbs, nobody ever sat down with him.

Jack pulled straight As that semester, and when he went home for the summer, Levon and Satenig could see the excitement on his face. Jack had found what he wanted to do. Everything he learned in his science classes seemed to open up new possibilities, and with that came a hunger for more knowledge. He told his parents he was planning on taking at least 30 credit hours the next semester, 10 more than was the norm, if the college would allow it.

His parents were certainly proud of Jack's accomplishments but his mother was concerned that he was working too hard and not participating in any of the campus enjoyment that university life offered. She especially wanted Jack to be more social and outgoing, perhaps even to have a girlfriend.

Although covertly wishing to have a female companion, Jack found most women incomprehensible. To him they seemed to blab about movies and clothes and silly stuff like that. He really didn't know how to approach them. If he had had the social graces to accompany his good looks, he may have had the pick of many a pretty co-ed. But in fact his demanding workload and failure to eat properly or exercise were beginning to diminish his appearance.

Jack didn't particularly care about how he looked – he believed people wasted far too much time primping. He had a simple wardrobe, mainly consisting of threadbare cardigans that he threw over whatever shirt he was wearing. He kept his hair short and shaved every day; expending any more energy on his appearance seemed unnecessary. He was going to be a scientist, after all, and since nobody ever bothered Einstein about his hair, he figured nobody would care if he wore the same cardigan a few days in a row. He was more interested in developing his mind than sacrificing study time just so he could have a more muscular physique. But at his mother's suggestion, Jack inspected himself in the mirror.

As he now looked at himself, Jack felt sick. Fat layered his face like strips of dough. A double chin had begun to develop. His skin was a ghostly white. He ran out of the bathroom in search of his mother's scales. Being small-boned and about 5'8" tall, his normal weight was about 120 pounds. When he stepped on the scales, the sad truth hit home. He had swollen to a gluttonous 162 pounds.

The summer of his sophomore year Levon moved Jack into a supervisory position at one of the sites. The clerical job gave Jack time to think. Seeing the way the extra weight had altered his appearance was unsettling. He didn't like the way he looked, but more importantly, neglecting his body meant he was neglecting his health. That was the important thing. How someone looked was ultimately irrelevant, but a healthy individual would live longer, and would be able to make intellectual contributions for a far longer time. If he was going to contribute to mankind, he had a responsibility to improve his physical well-being.

After reading numerous contradictory diet books, he decided

on a solution of his own. First, finding himself distracted by the thumping of his heart and the trembling of his hands, he set a limit of four cups of coffee per day. In order to lose weight, he decided to reduce the amount he ate, not the variety of foods. Each day in the canteen he would load up his plate, eat half portions and discard the rest.

He lost 20 pounds in the first three weeks. The diet worked, and it was easy to do, so what had started out as a routine of choice quickly became a habit. His father told him that it was wasteful to leave half his food on his plate with so many people starving in other parts of the world, but to Jack it seemed a bigger waste to allow himself to become 40 pounds overweight.

Exercise was next on his list of physical improvements. Since getting good grades was a much easier task than getting into shape, he decided that his schoolwork would have to take a back seat for a while. He began to cut a few afternoon classes and made his way to the weight room at the school gym. At first, the array of weight lifting routines and the variety of benches, bars and weights baffled him, so he stayed in a corner of the weight room and watched others exercise. As they struggled through their routines, Jack jotted notes on how much weight they used, how they lifted it, and what exercises they did as follow-up. He then developed his own routine.

Within one semester, he was pleased with the results. Aside from his bowed legs, he felt he looked much better. He could now do 50 push ups anywhere, at any time, without strain. And with 40 pounds of fat melted away, Jack felt like he had much more energy, even to study. The new routine of diet and exercise became a lifelong habit (he continued to exercise even in prison until ill health forced him to stop).

Now that Jack had finally developed the mental and physical discipline he strived for, he felt he was prepared for any challenge that could come his way.

The next challenge was how to get into medical school. He was advised to wait another year before applying, but he didn't see the point in delay even though he was one of 1,900 applicants vying for 150 positions. This only strengthened his resolve; he never doubted that he would get in.

Impressed with his grades, he was granted an admission interview even though he still had 33 credits to finish before he'd even meet their minimum requirements. When the interviewer expressed concerns that Jack might drop out of medicine as he had engineering, or might find the work too difficult, Jack replied that he was not a quitter, and would keep re-applying until he was accepted.

'You might think I'm cocky for saying this,' he said, 'but the reason seems obvious to me. I'm one of the smartest guys you'll ever see walk through your door, but I'm not doing this because of my ego. I'm doing this because medicine needs me. You let me get into medical school, and I'll prove it's the best decision you've ever made.'

A few months later, the acceptance letter arrived.

The Kevorkian family celebrated Jack's acceptance into medical school with a private family dinner, but within days the entire neighbourhood knew of the good news. Jack enjoyed being a minor celebrity. Some in high school had mocked his bookishness, and even kids at college had rolled their eyes when he said he'd rather spend his free time studying. But in the Kevorkians' working-class community, parents pointed Jack out to their kids as an example of what they could achieve if they worked hard, while the old Armenian men in the coffee shops proudly proclaimed that they had always known little Jack was a genius. Levon and Satenig, however, tempered their praise, telling Jack that the hardest work was ahead of him. While Jack's medical school acceptance seemed to them as momentous as their escape from Armenia, it was only a step in the right direction, not a guarantee that all life's problems were over.

Still, Jack entered medical school with a swagger, confident that he could handle anything thrown at him. The very set-up of a medical education excited him. In the next few years his instructors would teach him everything they knew about how the human body worked. No question would go unanswered, and his desire to study and research any issue presented in class was simply expected. He could learn as much as he wanted to, spending day and night in the library, and no one would think him strange. And, the better he did in his classes, the more likely his instructors would take him under their wing and reveal the magic of their personal research. Jack thought he was in paradise.

However, Jack's ideas of graduating at the top of his class faded quickly. Surrounded by others as ambitious and focused as himself, he soon learned that he couldn't expect to get the highest score in every class. With tests and classes hammering him like cannon fire, Jack had to focus on keeping up. There was no point in mastering the topic for one test if that meant he would fail all the other tests that week. He had to discipline his intellectual curiosity. There simply wasn't enough time to explore every fascinating titbit raised in class. With a balanced approach to studying for his classes, Jack settled into a comfortable routine. Though his first year went quickly and Jack passed all his subjects, he confided to his family that medical school was much more difficult than he had expected.

When he entered his second year of medical school, a pathology class buoyed his spirits. Pathology is the study of disease. Pathologists tend not to work with living patients, but with specimens of tissue or blood which are analysed in order to provide information that will benefit the patient. Pathologists also do autopsies on cadavers to find the cause of death. The pathology class was modelled after the courses given in the great German universities of the 19th century. Medicine had experienced some of its biggest advances in the 19th century thanks to the pioneering methods of the German pathologist Rudolf Virchow, who blended elements of dissection and microbiology in his efforts to unravel the mysteries he discovered on his microscope slides. The German model of medical education particularly appealed to Jack. Students were expected to remember vast tracts of research and theory, just as in other classes, but they were also encouraged to experiment and build on what they learned.

In Jack's other medical classes, the approach was far more conservative. Students absorbed the information as if they were little more than vessels to be filled. In his pathology class, however, his teachers praised him when he questioned the theories in the textbook, and suggested ways he could pull together research to prove his own. Jack loved the intellectual freedom, the feeling that he was part of a group of scientists intent on discovering new truths. He began to spend more of his time in the research lab, eager to follow in the trailblazing footsteps of the 19th century doctors and discover a breakthrough worthy of a Nobel Prize.

Jack's pathology class invigorated him. He felt like an investigator on the cutting edge of science, contributing to a body of knowledge that could improve the lives of everyone. Pathology was an all-encompassing discipline requiring knowledge in all branches of medicine, which meant to Jack a challenge and an opportunity for research. He decided that when the time came, he would select pathology as his specialisation. All the other medical disciplines seemed far less interesting, and Jack found himself doing little more than what was required in those classes. The thought of being the kind of doctor who memorised facts and regurgitated diagnoses learned in class was of little interest to him. Without research or hands-on investigation of the human body, being a doctor would be no different than being an engineer.

By his own admission, Jack was an exceptional student of pathology but only an average student in his other courses. When he graduated, in 1952, he had slipped to the middle of his class. It didn't particularly matter to Jack. He felt that if he needed knowledge from the other fields of medicine, he could always just pick up a book and cram in the information. Medical school had made him an expert in that kind of studying.

As he prepared for his internship at Henry Ford Hospital in Detroit, Jack wrote letters to family and friends. One letter that he sent to Flora, then living in Germany, still exists. She had attended the University of Michigan for a year, then married Hermann Holzheimer, a career German diplomat whom she met while he was studying postgraduate law at the university. The letter to Flora was filled with so many cartoon drawings that it seemed more a comic book than a loving letter to the sister he missed. He wrote that he was pleased that the hospital was close to home so he could be near his mother and father, and that he would finally be much less of a financial burden now that he was working. What Jack wrote most about, however, was his renewed interest in music, how it was becoming increasingly important to him. He was beginning to investigate opera, which he found fascinating, and was addicted to listening to Bach. It seemed as if he was far more eager to go to the opera than begin his internship.

Jack had trepidations about his first step in his medical career. The Henry Ford Hospital was one of the largest in the nation. A mere intern could be lost in the shuffle, limiting the amount of hands-on training he could receive. Instead of the training he craved, Jack settled for discussion with the senior doctors and doctors conducting independent research. He could only look on while senior staff members did the attendance. When he was allowed to directly involve himself in the treatment of patients, he was limited to drawing blood and inserting intravenous (IV) lines. Although he enjoyed the patient contact, the general setting was little different than the boring classrooms of medical school.

Feeling like an overqualified nurse, Jack tried to calm his frustrations by listening to music when he got home each evening, but images of some of the patients haunted him. In the paediatric unit he noticed a hydrocephalic boy strapped to a hospital bed and hooked to a ventilator. The birth defect had left him with an oversized, nearly boxlike head, the skull deformed by the pressure of the miasma of fluids that filled the space where his brain should have been. The boy would never wake, would never have a conscious thought, and yet the hospital kept him alive with feeding tubes and respirators. Jack felt it a disgusting waste of hospital resources, a violation of medical ethics. If doctors were supposed to act in their patients' best interests, it certainly seemed far more reasonable to let the boy die as nature had intended, rather than extend heroic efforts in preserving a brain-dead shell.

In another section of the hospital, Jack came across a cancer-ravaged woman. She was completely immobile, her jaundiced skin hanging off her bones. Her abdomen was stretched to five times its normal size by the fluids trapped within it, and the woman's face was frozen by the pain in what seemed to be a sardonic smile.

As Jack later wrote in his book *Prescription: Medicide*: 'It seemed as if she was pleading for help and death at the same time. Out of sheer empathy alone I could have helped her die with satisfaction. From that moment on, I was sure that doctor-assisted euthanasia and suicide are and always were ethical, no matter what anyone says or thinks.'

Jack had little time to explore this revelation, however. With the Korean War still raging as his internship finished, Jack volunteered his services to the military. The army ordered him to Texas for a month of special training as a first lieutenant medical officer and he was then flown to Eighth Army Headquarters in Seoul, Korea. Jack wasn't excited by the prospect of entering a war zone. His childhood fascination with stories of bullets and bravery had matured into a doctor's distaste for the butchery of war. But at least it would enable him to receive the hands-on experience that had been denied him during his internship.

When the military learned of Jack's fluency in Japanese, Jack had no hope of serving as an unnoticed doctor. The Koreans had been forced to learn Japanese from the time Japan occupied the country in 1905 to the end of World War II, and Japanese Kanji characters were also based on Chinese script, so Jack's knowledge of the language meant that he was suited to replace the Chinese-American captain who, after serving as the medical intelligence officer at headquarters, was returning to the US. Jack was often called upon to communicate with wounded Chinese soldiers trapped behind US lines, as well as to 'motivate' the Korean civilians assisting the US operation. When the Korean civilians were thought to be shirking their duties, Jack would sneak up behind them and bark orders in Japanese. Conditioned by years of Japanese occupation to immediately follow such orders or face the consequences, the Korean civilians rushed back to work.

Jack's superiors made ample use of his abilities in other ways. When the US attempted to exchange prisoners with the Chinese in Operation 'Big Switch' in 1954, they called on Jack to assist in negotiations. When one of the Chinese Colonels insisted on addressing the finer points of the compromise in German, Jack was able to fill the void and translated for the American officers.

When the military weren't making use of his language skills, Jack spent half of each day handling 'sick call' in the base medical clinic and coordinated the preventative medical activities of the units stationed near the Demilitarised zone. Despite the responsibilities placed upon him, Jack felt constrained. The translation work was interesting, and the medical work gave him valuable experience, but it all too quickly became a mindless routine. He longed to return to the US and pursue research.

To ease the boredom, Jack and other doctors walked through the surrounding cratered hills, pausing occasionally to investigate the unburied old skeletons of enemy soldiers. When an acquaintance died after stumbling over a landmine, however, the military insisted that Jack remain on base. Trapped in the barracks complex, and feeling isolated from the other men by his position and responsibilities, Jack wiled away the time learning to read and write Latin and Greek. When even that began to bore him, Jack turned to playing Bach on his flute, the lilting notes softening the chill of the lonely, freezing winter.

After 15 months in Korea, Jack was ordered to report to Camp Hale in Colorado to serve as the medical officer during training operations for the mountain and ski troops. The position required him to spend many freezing nights in a sleeping bag and tent 14,000 feet up a mountain, but Jack relished the chilling beauty of the mountains since he knew that he would only have to serve a few more months in the military. He enjoyed tramping through the snow, which at times stood as much as 15 feet deep, and he devised a relatively accurate way to guess the temperature of the air from the squeaking of the snow under his feet as he walked.

Though he no longer witnessed the battlefield injuries of soldiers carted in for medical care, the memory of what he had seen in Korea began to haunt his thoughts. So many soldiers had simply bled to death because the army's blood supply couldn't reach them in time. Others had lingered in pain, suffering through amputations and surgeries that only marginally lengthened their already shattered lives. There had to be ways to address such issues. He promised himself he would find solutions when he had the time to investigate the problems at his own leisure.

In June 1955 Jack was finally released from active duty. He returned home to begin his first year of residency in pathology at the University of Michigan Medical Center, eager to begin research. The hospital administrators, however, had different plans for him. Like most residents, he was considered highly trained, but inexpensive, help. Since Jack needed additional experience and study before being allowed to practise medicine unsupervised, he was assigned the preparatory work that the staff doctors detested. Soon his days were filled with autopsies and the preparation of surgical specimens for diagnosis, but Jack made free time to investigate the old medical journals kept in the hospital library. In his autopsy work, Jack was curious as to why the time of death was always considered an approximation. The time of death was usually placed within an hour of when rigor mortis had set in, but that seemed more like guesswork than a scientific method.

In one of the old journals, Jack uncovered an obscure mid-19th century French study. The doctors at the time recognised that the retinas in patients' eyes contracted when they were near death, and using the newly invented ophthalmoscope, they tried to record images of the retinas of dying patients in order to provide a more accurate way to determine death. At the time, the big concern was with preventing people from being buried alive, and so the doctors were only concerned with finding out if the dilation of the retina was directly linked to whether or not a person was still alive.

Jack thought the experiment could go further. If he could duplicate their experiments while meticulously recording the changes to the retina, he was sure that he could not only show whether or not a person was dead, but pinpoint exactly when they died. His theory could assist pathologists, forensic psychiatrists, and police forces in solving homicides and convicting the perpetrators. He mentioned his theory to the chief of pathology and was given permission to proceed.

After getting the consent of the families of the patients and the ward doctors responsible for the patients' care, Jack pursued his research every free moment. Carting along an electrocardiogram and a small camera, Jack set up his equipment beside the patients.

66

When the electrocardiogram indicated that a patient's heart was about to stop, Jack taped open their eyes and snapped a series of photographs. Jack and his camera became a frequent sight in many of the wards.

The nurses, however, had little idea what the young resident was doing. They knew that he was researching death, and felt that what he was doing was unnatural – and creepy. Soon the staff took to referring to the young resident's research as 'the doctor of death's death rounds'. Within a few months, they simply began referring to him as Dr Death. The nickname stuck.

Though the research struck many as irrelevant and bizarre, it was groundbreaking work. Jack meticulously recorded his findings, detailing how the retina expanded and contracted near death, how its colour slowly shifted from the brightness of life to a pale orange-red, then yellow and finally grey. The purpose of measuring exact time of death could probably have been most beneficial in forensics, for criminal investigations. Jack, through experience and research, was able to predict time of death within one half-hour 79 per cent of the time, and within ten minutes 29 per cent of the time. Had further research been done and the results taught in college, it may have helped emergency medical technicians to know when it was still possible to save a patient and when it was not, and to develop standards for instituting heroic measures. Unfortunately, the research was never picked up or expanded upon.

Jack wrote an article about his findings titled 'The Fundus Oculi and the Determination of Death' for the *American Journal of Pathology*. When it was published, Jack felt like a real researcher poised to make valuable contributions to mankind. He was certain others would recognise the merit of his work and ask for him to push forward. Nobody did, and his conclusive methodology is shunned to this day.

Still, Jack was intent on pursuing research. At the end of his first year of residency, he travelled to Germany to visit Flora. While there, he met a local cardiac surgeon from the Kranken-haus en ber Isar hospital in Munich, who allowed Jack to sit in during open-heart surgeries. Though he wasn't allowed to bring a camera into the operating room with him, Jack put his drawing skills to use and sketched the patients' retinas at the moment the cardiac surgeon cut off blood circulation to perform the surgery. He wrote up his findings and published his research in a German journal, then joined in with a researcher investigating the pineal gland, an organ of the brain that secretes the pigmentation hormone melatonin, and wrote an article on that as well.

By the time his stay in Germany drew to a close, Jack was a fully fledged researcher with published articles, although he hadn't even finished his residency. He decided that when he returned to the US he would pursue research even more vigorously. He wasn't interested in joining the research studies already in progress at the hospital, as they seemed only minor extensions of unimportant work. He wanted to find something to research on his own, a project full of risks and real rewards.

Chapter 5

NOTORIETY

Jack returned from Germany ready to move forward with his research. He eagerly told the other residents about the work he had seen researchers performing in the German universities. He hoped that some of the residents at the hospital had noticed his articles, but if any of them had they didn't mention it. When he discussed his research and how much it energised him, the other residents only smiled. While he had been gone, a number of them had begun to ponder whether or not it might have been better if Dr Death stayed in Germany. His bizarre experiments certainly weren't going to make them, or their hospital, look good in the public eye, with their national colleagues or with the American Medical Association (AMA). Their duty, as they saw it, was to conduct reasonable research on disease and the cures for disease in order to save lives. Staring into a dead man's eyeballs was not normal, and whatever it was that Jack thought he was learning by doing so didn't seem to them to be of any benefit to the medical community. At best he was a harmless nut, but at worst he could damage the reputation of the hospital, and that could hurt their careers.

They urged him to look into topics with more practical use, such as some upcoming drug studies. Jack, however, was not interested in looking at slides all day, going over blood and tissue samples. The other residents told Jack that his few published papers didn't give him licence to do as he pleased.

Jack was furious. The residents acknowledged that he was a good researcher, but they seemed jealous of his success. It was clear to Jack that he was the only one doing anything innovative. The other residents talked about their work helping in the battle against death, but he was actually exploring death itself in a way no one else had ever done before.

Jack craved the respect of the other residents even while knowing it was foolhardy to expect them to come around to his way of thinking. They were a part of a system that pumped out doctors every year, training them to follow the established guidelines of medicine. It was an inherently conservative system that advocated restraint and caution. For them, it was far better to follow a procedure known to be only marginally effective than to try something new. Being a doctor shielded them from personal responsibility for the deaths that accrued. When a treatment failed, they could always say that they had done the best that medicine allowed. Rather than devise new treatments or risk a new procedure, they turned to the hierarchy of medicine. Medical students consulted interns, interns consulted residents and residents were expected to turn to senior staff. The assumption was that the longer you practised medicine, the more you knew, and the better you were equipped to handle the tough decisions. It didn't matter if the senior staff were out of touch with modern practices and maintained the status quo, one simply didn't buck the system.

One hospital ritual Jack dreaded was the weekly departmental teaching session in the autopsy room. Attendance was mandatory, and the residents were expected to listen to the lectures of senior staff, then summarise cases and accurately pinpoint and discuss the progress of a disease using tissue samples. The sessions weren't much different from many of his medical school classes. A senior staff member would have them look at a slide under a microscope, or gather around an examination table to look at a prepared organ sample, then pepper them with basic questions about what they had seen. The doctor in charge would keep at it until they had regurgitated the pertinent information. It seemed to Jack to be more like a weekly pop quiz on pathology than real training.

During one of these sessions, however, a resident raised a question that piqued Jack's interest. The doctor in charge had just finished a dry lecture on autopsy procedures and asked if anyone had any questions. The residents blearily looked up, baffled. They had already known the procedures the doctor had discussed, and had, in fact, been using them for months. The only real question, Jack thought, was why they were being forced to waste time going over something they had already proven they knew. Of course, if they didn't ask a question the doctor would think they hadn't been paying attention, and eventually some senior staff member would arrange a teaching session to go over the issue again.

The silence seemed to last minutes. Finally a resident raised his hand and asked how the current autopsy procedures came into being. The doctor in charge wasn't familiar with the history of autopsy, nor could he point to any reading material on the subject, and he suggested the residents focus purely on current techniques. Jack interjected, stating that there was actually a lot written on the subject – but that it was in German. The doctor challenged Jack to do some research and prove to him how knowing the history of autopsy would be any more relevant to medicine than Jack's studies of corpses' retinas.

The residents laughed, and Jack felt a flush rising in his face. The doctor expected him to back down, but Jack was never one to run from adversity.

During his free time, Jack looked through the large medical library in the hospital in search of answers. Though a number of books were full of useful information on current treatments, very few touched on anything earlier than the 20th century, so he began searching through German language publications. Jack asked the medical librarian to help by getting copies of the journals he had been reading in Germany.

The details about the Alexandrians were nebulous. There weren't many documents about their experiments, but he came across criticisms of the Alexandrian's work written by Roman historians 400 years after the fact. That meant that dissection was at least 2,200 years old. And from what he read, it became clear that although modern techniques of dissection were recent innovations, they had been evolving for nearly as long as Western civilisation.

Jack presented his findings on the history of the autopsy during the next departmental teaching session and was greeted with a stunned silence. He rapidly covered the slow evolution of techniques, the stops and starts as taboos came into play. The church had been a major influence in slowing the pace of research, prohibiting researchers from acquiring cadavers or doing any inspection that was more than skin deep. For centuries researchers had done the work in secret and as a result their findings were not publicised, so others had to learn their processes anew. The best developers of dissection technique were afraid to talk about what they did, and so their skills died with them. Many made use of grave robbers to supply them with research cadavers, but Jack came across a few rumoured incidents of experiments being conducted on the living. In those cases, consent was rarely given. The victim of the experiments was often a slave or a prisoner, someone who had little chance of escaping their fate. Jack traced the history of autopsy through the centuries and concluded by saying, 'A lot of you have been saying that I must be obsessed with death. If so, I'm just following a tradition set down for researchers like us by the Greeks and others. And if you still wonder why I do the research I do, you should understand now. Our predecessors wanted to completely understand the human body, but they were never allowed to. They committed crimes in order to do their research, and they often made so many mistakes that their research was useless. Yet, what they were trying to piece together is exactly what we're dedicated to as well. All I'm doing is taking up the torch, but this time, I'll make sure we do things right.'

The other residents applauded when he was done, and even the chief of the department, Dr James A French, vigorously shook Jack's hand. He felt the material should be published. He warned Jack that he was dealing with some powerful taboos and should be careful, but he assured him that he would help smooth the way with his paper.

Though he'd delved into other journals during his research, Jack kept returning to the article on the Alexandrians. During that time, the Hellenistic Greek scientists had been just as fascinated with determining the line between life and death as he was, despite facing similar hostilities. It seemed as if it was human nature to reject such experiments, as if the very mention of dissection triggered an instinctive desire to protect the body. As a result, during the time of the Alexandrians there was no way for them to investigate the workings of the human body. They didn't have anaesthetics so it was impossible to recruit live volunteers. The bodies of the dead were off limits as well. Ptolemy, however, had permitted medical experiments on criminals condemned to death. If not for the Alexandrian ruler's decree that condemned criminals would be executed by submitting to the experiments of the scientists, anatomy would have remained a complete mystery for millennia.

Jack later said that discovering the article on the Alexandrians was a turning point in his career. As he pondered what the Alexandrians had achieved, he realised that not only were they the originators of modern autopsies, but they had also provided a reasonable method for pursuing medical research on the human body. Though now cadavers are donated for research purposes, it is still impossible to perform research on living bodies. Using convicts scheduled to receive the death penalty could change all that.

Jack wasn't oblivious to the potential problems, but he felt that others would recognise how valuable the work could be to medicine. The Alexandrians hadn't given the convicts any choice in the matter. They had simply picked out the convicts they wanted for research, and then forced them to drink themselves into an alcoholic coma before they began cutting into them. Modern doctors wouldn't have to resort to such barbarism. First, Jack felt the decision to be a part of such research should be something the convicts voluntarily made for themselves. Though they were convicts, they were still human beings, and it was important that any scientist respect the personal autonomy of the convict. Second, the best in modern anaesthesia should be made available to the convict during the procedure so he wouldn't experience any pain.

Jack was not in favour of the death penalty, but felt that if the state was going to take a life, some good might as well come of it. Death penalty laws could be adjusted to grant the condemned on death row a choice between the conventional methods of execution and the Alexandrian form of medical experimentation. If the convict wanted to be a part of the research, then irreversible surgical depth anaesthesia would be induced at the exact instant set for execution. Once the experiments were done, an executioner could administer a final overdose of anaesthesia. The convict would feel no pain, they would avoid a meaningless death and the research would tremendously advance the cause of medicine. It seemed like a perfect idea.

This was, of course, long before lethal injection became the standard method of capital punishment in the United States (Oklahoma first adopted this means of execution in 1977, but it wasn't until 1982 that it was used). At the time, most convicts who were executed were sent to the electric chair, while others were hanged or faced a firing squad, all violent and painful methods of dying. To Jack's way of thinking – which he later admitted 'reeked with sophomoric idealism and was highly impractical' – it seemed more humane to put prisoners peacefully to sleep and use their bodies for a purpose that would end up benefiting the rest of mankind.

Jack desperately wanted to share his plan for using death row inmates in medical research with Dr French. But he stopped himself, it was too early. He still needed to work out all the details for his proposal, and, most importantly, he still had to sample the opinions of those on death row so he could offer evidence that condemned criminals supported the idea and would volunteer. He asked for, and was granted, a few days off to do more research.

A week later, on a crisp and sunny October day, Jack drove his light blue, two-door 56 Ford south on I-75 towards Columbus, Ohio. Michigan had a moratorium on capital punishment so the Ohio Penitentiary was the nearest death row. Jack knew little about how the prison system worked, who he would need to talk to or even where exactly the prison was, but he drove with the excitement of a man on a mission.

When he reached the penitentiary Jack began to have second thoughts. Surveying the iron bars, the sharp razor wire, the slits in the concrete that served as windows for the prison cells, he felt a great sadness come over him. How could anyone have any dignity in such a place? No rehabilitation could possibly go on in there.

Jack thought about why he was there and the value of what he was trying to do. If he did nothing, nothing would change. Executions would continue, their only result being the destruction of one life as an attempt to appease those who had suffered at the criminal's hands. But if Jack made it possible for prisoners to volunteer their bodies in the service of science, he would be giving those men a little of their dignity back. Those who wanted to see them dead would still get their wish and vengeance would wreak its terrible price. At the same time, however, the prisoner would be given a meaningful way to at least partially repay his debt to society. What if a better method of open-heart surgery was discovered while working on a convict? What if a scientist tried a radical form of brain surgery on a prisoner, free of the fears associated with making a mistake during surgery, and discovered a new method that saved lives? Jack felt he had a responsibility; he had to have the courage to walk through the front doors and see if any prisoners were willing to join him on his mission.

That didn't keep Jack's hands from shaking as he entered the prison. The Spartan concrete walls seemed to close in around him. He could barely splutter out his reason for visiting the prison when he reached the front desk and had to show his identification card to prove that he really was a doctor. Finally, after nearly an hour spent leaning against a wall near the front desk, a guard directed him towards the warden's office.

The warden, Ralph Alvis, was a husky, balding man who stared icily at Jack and scolded him for not knowing the penitentiary's visitation rules. Jack pleaded to be heard.

Fully expecting to get kicked out at any moment, Jack hurried through an impromptu speech. He mentioned the hospital, his research, the Alexandrians, the benefits of studying live bodies. While he had been driving from Michigan, he had imagined himself delivering the same speech with far more control and authority. Instead, faced with the stony, unemotional silence of the warden, Jack found himself babbling.

But to Jack's surprise, Alvis seemed sympathetic to his cause. He told Jack that he had just visited his father, who was suffering from heart problems, in the hospital. There wasn't anything doctors could do to save his father's life. But if Jack's idea worked, maybe there would be some way one of the convicts could help his dad or others like him.

He agreed to do what he could to help, and asked a guard to take Jack to death row to talk to some prisoners.

Jack could barely contain his excitement. They had only talked for a few minutes, and without any paperwork or bureaucratic hassle the warden had given him the OK for what was, without a doubt, the cornerstone of his plan.

The guard led Jack out the rear exit of Alvis' office and through a maze of cellblocks and windowless corridors until they reached a thick metal door. They squeezed past into a 5-foot square cubicle composed of heavy steel plates, and only after the door clanged behind them, and the guard had tapped in what seemed like Morse code on the cubicle wall with his night stick, did the door to death row open.

As Jack surveyed death row, the uneasiness that had temporarily paralysed him in the parking lot returned. The lighting was dim and flickered like candlelight. Along one wall was a row of small cells, each barred by a thick steel gate covered in a screen of steel wire. He had expected to hear chatter as he entered death row, perhaps even a few taunting inmates, but he was greeted only by silence, as if, he thought, the men within the cells were already dead.

The guard set out two stools in front of one of the cells. He motioned Jack onto one, then opened the door to the cell and guided a young, muscular white man to the other stool. Jack and the convict stared at each other. Jack wasn't sure where to begin. It was one thing to describe how his plan would work and to ponder the possibilities, quite another to be faced with the task of telling a death row inmate, a man with a known history of murder, that he wanted to dissect and experiment on him – to cut him up before he was executed! It wasn't something they had taught him in medical school.

Jack searched for a euphemism for the execution the convict faced. He wanted to broach the subject in a sensitive way. Finally, after moments of silence, Jack stammered, 'You know why you're here,' in a staccato outburst.

The convict kept staring at him, his face a cold mask.

Jack told the prisoner that he was not there to help him, but rather to show him how he might be of help to others.

The convict furrowed his brow and cocked his head. Jack had his attention. With renewed confidence, he explained why he had come to the penitentiary and what he hoped to do. The convict listened politely, nodding from time to time. When Jack finished, the condemned man looked up at the guard and told him that by doing this, it was possible that science could learn something from his body that might help his little daughter in the future.

He was not only interested, he wanted to sign up immediately, and asked Jack what he had to do to get started. Jack replied, 'Just write me a letter putting your opinion in writing.'

The other convicts that Jack interviewed were less open to the idea. One, a young black man who had murdered a policeman, admitted that Jack's plan sounded like a good one, but he wasn't willing to commit himself to it without first talking it over with his wife and his father, who was a Baptist minister. He eventually sent a letter saying that he wanted to postpone his decision but Jack never heard from him again. The other prisoners that Jack talked to were reticent to put their opinions in writing. They looked at Jack warily, unwilling to trust him.

When Jack drove back towards Ann Arbor, however, he was elated. He hadn't expected every inmate to agree to his plan, but he had hoped to find at least one that did. He now also had a clearer sense of the obstacles he faced. The plan might be a good one, but not every prisoner was going to accept it, and some would be too suspicious of him to even hear him out. That wouldn't matter in the long run though. All he needed to get to the next step of his plan was proof that at least one prisoner was willing to donate his body for experimentation. He was sure that once that prisoner's execution day came along, and the other prisoners saw how he had been treated and the good that had come of his volunteering, they would spontaneously volunteer as well.

When he arrived home, Jack began writing an essay outlining his proposal and suggesting how best for it to be implemented. He started by stating his neutrality on the concept of capital punishment. Personally, he didn't see the point or purpose in capital punishment in the first place, but that was irrelevant to his proposal. Capital punishment was a reality in many states, and so the best thing he could do would be to provide a more rational, humane, compassionate and beneficial way to carry it out. Ideally, in Jack's way of thinking, anyone condemned to death should be allowed the choice to be executed by the method prescribed by law, or by controlled general anaesthesia after they had been used for medical experimentation. Everyone who participated in the medical experimentation procedure would have to do so by their own choice, even the scientists involved, without coercion. Any proposed research would need to be approved by an international panel, perhaps a body of scientists within the United Nations. They would approve the experiment; the scientists involved, the prisoner involved, and ensure that an appropriate laboratory was being used for the purpose.

While Jack was writing his proposal, a letter came to him in the mail. It was from the first man he had interviewed on death row. The proof that prisoners could agree to his proposal was finally in his hands, and Jack carefully put it in a folder. The letter, he felt, needed to be shared with others because of how eloquently the prisoner had stated his own feelings on the procedure.

I feel the same today as I did yesterday when you asked me. I would gladly give you what you requested of me and in doing so it might help others in many years to come and quite possibly even now.

It would also help me to think that I didn't succeed in making a total mess of my life, that I may have helped someone, somewhere, sometime.

I don't want you to think that I'm a brave man or a hero because that would be wrong, but if I must die, I must, but your way would be much more humane and at the same time beneficial to others.

The prisoner's letter spurred Jack to quickly complete his proposal. As he wrote, he pondered what must have been going through the convict's mind, if the compassion that seemed evident in the letter had always been a part of him or if it was something new that had come upon him while he was on death row. Jack thought that his proposal might actually help scientists understand the criminal mind and how it operated. What if, by studying a convict's brain, they discovered abnormal physiology that had led to him committing murder in the first place? In the future, doctors could spot such issues and surgically correct them, preventing criminal behaviour. Or what if the issues were due to a chemical imbalance that only became apparent when investigating a living brain? Again, the possibilities seemed endless. The brain was the greatest mystery facing scientists, and yet scientists were prevented from studying one while alive. Instead, they were expected to make educated guesses based on animal brains, or based on what they had uncovered from a cold, inert human brain during autopsy. The taboo against working with a living brain made scientists as ineffective as blindfolded men trying to describe the colour and texture of a Pollock painting.

Overflowing with excitement, Jack rushed to the hospital to show his essay to Dr French. Though the doctor was in his office talking to a few other residents, Jack decided no one would mind if he walked right in. After all, the head of the department had given him permission to take a few days off to continue his research, and he had even mentioned that he was aware of the taboos Jack faced and was eager to smooth the way for him. But when Jack walked in, he felt everyone in the room was irritated with him before he even spoke.

When Jack explained that he had his paper done, the chief told him just to leave it on his desk. Jack, however, insisted that he needed to explain some of his ideas that might not have been made clear in his rush to get the paper done. The chief objected, saying he was sure he could understand anything Jack had written about the history of autopsy. 'This isn't that essay,' said Jack. 'This is a new research proposal. For performing experiments on death row inmates.'

Jack quickly recapped his proposal and what he had encountered on his trip to Ohio. After a few sentences, the doctor had seated himself at his desk, a look of incredulous disbelief on his face. The other doctors in the room were equally stunned. One of the residents remarked that they were not in Nazi Germany, after all. Jack couldn't understand the comparison. This was different – this was not cruel experimentation on innocent victims, this would be done with the convicts' consent.

The department chief argued that Jack's experiments would go against the Hippocratic oath, and warned Jack that he would be throwing away his medical career if he pursued this idea any further. He would not lend Jack his support.

'I don't need it,' Jack said, and stridently left the office.

When Jack went home and thought over the confrontation, he had to admit that his essay was a bit idealistic. In order for his plan to work, a lot of prevailing notions of right and wrong would need readjustment, and that kind of social change didn't happen overnight or simply because someone wanted the world to change. Still, he believed in his idea. Practical or not, it had real potential and shouldn't be abandoned just because others were afraid of it. He concluded that there was nothing else to do but push the issue as far as he could. He would shoot for the moon. He quickly edited the essay, deciding not to compromise on any points, and titled it 'Capital Punishment or Capital Gain'.

During the next few weeks he submitted the article to several medical journals and popular magazines, but was roundly rejected at every step. He believed his idea might get more support if people actually heard it, so he contacted the chairman of the Criminology Section of the American Association for the Advancement of Science. They were scheduled to have their annual meeting that December and Jack felt that this meeting would provide the perfect forum for discussing his ideas – but by this time he expected his paper to be rejected out of hand. Surprisingly, his paper was accepted immediately.

The events surrounding the presentation of his paper were to radically change Jack's life. Only later did he realise that the chairman, a vociferous opponent of capital punishment, hoped that Jack's paper would horrify others and garner more support for the chairman's allies. At the time, all Jack cared about was that the public would finally hear his ideas. The days until the meeting in December slipped by quickly.

When Jack went to Washington DC to present his paper, he was an unknown to everyone but his family, friends, co-workers and the few people who'd read his published articles. By the time the meeting was over, his name and his proposal were front-page news. The reaction to his presentation surprised everyone. The listening audience bombarded him with questions as soon as he was finished, but it was the local evening and weekend newspapers, who thought of the story as a strange piece about another crazy doctor, who really popularised him. Their accounts spread like wildfire through the wire services. Unfortunately, the debate Jack anticipated never materialised. The medical community was willing to write him off as a nutcase, while those on both sides of the capital punishment debate shied away rather than risk being associated with him.

However the *Journal of Criminal Law, Criminology, and Police Science* offered to publish his article, giving a needed and respected forum for his ideas. As well, a professor of sociology in the audience who had been conducting research on non-condemned prisoners in his state's penitentiary volunteered to help Jack pull together more prisoner opinions on Jack's plan. As Jack returned home, he felt positive about the whole experience. Not everyone had accepted his ideas, but people were beginning to listen. It was a start he could build on.

When he returned to the hospital, Jack was told to meet with Dr French for an important talk. He was excited to be able to relay all that had happened to him in Washington. Jack had created quite a stir. His ideas were now national news, and that could only be good for the hospital.

But when he entered into the department head's office, there was a cold stillness to the air, and the department head wasn't smiling. Despite that fact that he admired Jack's courage in saying what he believed, he gave Jack an ultimatum: quit the death penalty work or leave the residency programme.

As Jack walked through the hospital that day, saying quiet farewells to the hallways he had come to know so well, he felt a touch of sadness. At the same time, it was clear that he had made the right choice. He could always find another hospital. It was far better to do that than to keep quiet about his convictions. He had a responsibility to keep fighting; to himself, to his parents, to the teachers that believed in him and to medicine.

Jack, now in his early thirties, was pleased to find a hospital in his home town. Pontiac General eagerly welcomed Jack into its medical staff. Though he joked with his family that he had only been hired because doctors were in short supply, the truth was that good pathologists didn't just walk through the doors of Pontiac General every day. During the interview, Jack mentioned that he planned on pushing his research further. The administrators told him that as long as he attended to his duties in the pathology department, they wouldn't mind what he did with his spare time.

His fellow doctors didn't particularly care what he did either. When he mentioned his research to the other doctors in the staff lounge, the most common response was, 'You have time for research?' They were doctors fully engaged in practising medicine. Real research was something that happened elsewhere, far away from the trenches of a busy city hospital, performed by PhDs in lab coats. That Jack had done research on the retinas of the dead and had chatted with death row inmates fascinated them. His research sounded a bit bizarre, but it had more practical value than most of the studies they saw filling the pages of medical journals.

At first, Jack considered returning to his death row plan. When his name had first hit the headlines after he attended the conference in Washington DC, he had been contacted by the chairman of a special committee in Ohio. They were considering revisions to the state's death penalty laws. Jack had prepared a packet containing copies of his essay and several supportive letters from other researchers and theologians, and he handed the material out when he met the committee members. At first the members were sceptical, but Jack was so focused on his idea, and oblivious to their reaction, that his passionate plea lasted nearly 20 minutes. A front-page story in the local paper the next day quoted a legislator as having said that he first thought Jack was a crackpot, but that he had changed his mind after listening to his presentation. Another legislator said that he was so impressed that he wanted to introduce a bill to assist Jack's efforts.

Jack didn't believe the death penalty provided society any positive benefits, but he had hoped that, if society was adamant about killing its convicts, it would at least attempt to gain some benefit from their deaths by allowing them to volunteer for research. He quickly realised, however, that such efforts were ill timed. This was the early 60s; public sentiment had been steadily turning against capital punishment, and his efforts in support of his death row plan could be mistakenly construed as support for the death penalty. That was the last thing he wanted. He therefore no longer actively pursued the death row plan.

Jack would later say that the best times of his life were at Pontiac General. He now worked near his parent's home, so he frequently dropped in to check on them and make sure they were doing OK. The family often gathered there for big Sunday dinners. Although Flora was away travelling the world with her husband, Margo (who had been married and divorced) and her daughter were there every week. Aside from needling him to get married soon, his parents were pleased with how Jack had turned out, and they were glad to see him so happy at the hospital. The other doctors saw Jack as down to earth, and even funny. He fitted right in. They accepted Jack and his research, and although Jack would never have publicly admitted it, their acceptance gave him renewed confidence. He began to let his guard down, and started to develop genuine friendships.

One of those friendships was with the gregarious Neal Nicol, a man who would become Jack's right-hand man and loyal friend for decades to come.

Neal was surprised to see Dr Kevorkian carrying his lunch tray over to the table Neal was sharing with some other medical technicians. Neal had seen Jack in the halls of the hospital, but they had only discussed test results of lab work for which Neal was responsible. Neal hadn't bothered trying to have a personal conversation because he felt doctors usually thought their medical degree meant they should be treated like royalty, and if they actually learned your name it was only a matter of time before they began to order you around like their personal servant.

The medical technicians had been taking turns telling jokes between bites of lunch, and Neal had just finished one that he said he heard during his three-year hitch overseas. The laughter at the table died when Jack walked up.

Neal pointed to the other end of the cafeteria, and told Jack that's where the doctors were sitting. Jack said he'd rather sit with a group of people whose laughter he could hear from across the room. When Neal said he was afraid that Jack night be offended by their raunchy humour, Jack replied that he was offended only by stupidity – and that he had raunchy jokes of his own. Neal then commented that nothing could top the jokes he'd heard while serving in Japan, and the men realised they had their military service in common.

While the rest of the table quickly resumed its chatter, the two men reminisced about their time serving the military. They also discovered they were both Michigan kids born into working-class families, and though their lives had taken them along different educational paths, they shared a similar working-class no-nonsense approach to living life. As they talked, the invisible barrier that existed between doctors and the other staff slowly disappeared. They were like two neighbourhood kids hanging out on a street corner, trying to one-up each other with stories that were part joke, part tall tale.

And yet if it hadn't been for the military their lifelong friendship would never have been possible. When Neal graduated from his Detroit high school in 1957, he enlisted in the army like many other kids in his neighbourhood had done. He hadn't been sure of what he wanted to do after high school, and the army seemed to provide a number of opportunities. For a working-class kid without any real plan for the future, entering the military was a logical step. Since he was enlisting instead of being forced into service by the draft, he was given a choice as to the career training he would receive in the military.

He thought that being a medical technician sounded interesting. He could see himself in a bright white lab coat, bustling about with beakers and vials, examining slides under a microscope and chasing nurses. That was a job that would turn heads in the neighbourhood.

As his tour of duty drew to a close, he began to feel that being a medical technician might not be such a bad thing. He could see himself doing the same work back home, pulling in a regular pay cheque while saving himself from the tedious work on the assembly line, where many of the other kids from his working-class neighbourhood were destined. When he returned to the US in 1961 and joined Pontiac General, it was with a renewed optimism about what his life could be.

By the time Neal met Jack, he had come to accept the fact that his work at the hospital would only rarely challenge him. The life of a medical technician wasn't nearly as exciting as he had imagined when the army recruiter had first mentioned it, but at least it was steady if boring work. He took pride in knowing that what he did was helping patients, but the longer he worked in the hospital, the less respect he had for the doctors. The doctors treated him like an invisible, unimportant functionary of the hospital.

Not every doctor was incompetent, but as far as Neal knew they were all unwilling to admit when they were unsure of what they were doing, and pathologically incapable of asking anyone other than another doctor for advice or assistance with their diagnoses. They were also terrified they would be requested to testify in court regarding a blood or tissue sample they had interpreted. Neal knew he had problems dealing with authority, but he felt his opinion of doctors was completely justified.

As he got to know Jack, however, his opinion slowly changed. During lunch the two would banter until it was time to get back to work, ribbing each other about the women that caught their eye, spinning jokes or trying to nail down why the culture they had come across in Korea and Japan seemed so alien to the one found in America. Their search for girlfriends was a common point of discussion and an easy way for Neal to tease Jack. Jack was spectacularly unsuccessful at cultivating a long-term relationship with a member of the opposite sex. Sometimes the two of them would spot the same woman and talk about how they were going to approach her, but it was inevitably Neal who worked up the courage to ask women out on dates. Jack, on occasion, was able to get a date as well, and sometimes the two of them would double date, but it was more common for him to be on his own than in the company of a woman. Whenever Neal asked him what had gone wrong, Jack would answer with one of two basic responses: either they had argued and the woman had impulsively decided to end it, or they had argued and Jack had decided against pursuing the relationship. 'I just haven't found the right woman yet,' Jack would say, to which Neal could reply, 'Maybe I could loan you some of mine.'

Jack was unlike the other doctors. He recognised that he was an exceptionally gifted doctor, and he took pride in his skills, but if a nurse or a technician had a suggestion he would listen and either implement their suggestions or explain why their suggestions wouldn't work. And though Jack was a confident and self-assured man, he wasn't afraid to make a self-deprecating remark if that would get someone to laugh. He took his work seriously but not himself, and that, as far as Neal was concerned, was the way a doctor should be.

Jack began to include Neal as a willing accomplice in his plans, just as he had with the neighbourhood kids in his youth. Neal was interested in the research Jack had done, and his frequent praise and encouragement of Jack's efforts, as well as his obvious skill as a medical technician, made the union a practical one.

Their first scheme together had the best intentions, and was great fun, but the results were less than perfect. It started from a discussion they'd had about how frightened patients were when they came into the hospital. It distressed Jack that the public had so many misconceptions about what they would face when they walked into a hospital. He was stunned at how often patients and their families balked at simple procedures. In 1961, many people still had the view of hospitals as places where sick people go to die. Few of today's life-saving drugs and surgical procedures existed, and most hospital staff had little or no training in how to treat incoming patients.

Jack and another doctor on staff, Shelby Baylis, whom Jack knew from medical school, enlisted Neal to help make a training film that could allay the concerns of new patients while also educating staff about what patients faced. A film could make the hospital professionals more aware of the need for compassion, and encourage them to spend more time attempting to ease patient fears.

Jack rented a 16mm black and white camera, and they began sketching out what the film would cover. As their plan coalesced, Jack approached the hospital administrators and told them what the movie was all about. They told him that they would likely have no problem with the film being shown to the rest of the staff and to incoming patients whenever possible. Encouraged by their support, Jack then approached the owner of the downtown Pontiac Theater and convinced him to debut the movie when it was completed. Jack's excitement was contagious. He thought it was possible that the film could get screened at other hospitals and at bigger theatres. He imagined it making its way across the country; subtly influencing the way patients and doctors came together.

Jack and Shelby began filming as soon as they figured out how the camera worked. Shelby played a garbage collector with a sudden attack of appendicitis. Jack acted as the attending ER physician. Neal had a bit part as a recuperating occupational rehabilitation patient. The film was simply structured: one scene presented the ER encounter the way the garbage collector viewed it, while the other presented the encounter as it would actually happen in a hospital setting. The first scene seemed as if it was pulled directly from a horror movie. The poor garbage collector wandered in complaining of abdominal pain, only to be promptly whisked into surgery and, effectively, butchered by the overeager doctor who believed that the only way to correctly diagnose a problem was to keep cutting through the body until you found the source of pain. In the second scene, the patient was led through a series of innocuous blood draws and tests until the problem was isolated, and then operated on quickly and efficiently after the situation had been fully explained. Filmed in grainy black and white by the shaky and inexperienced hands of Jack, Shelby and Neal, the movie was humorous and informative, but definitely of amateur quality. The hospital administrators backed off when they saw it.

Still, Jack attended the premiere at the Pontiac Theater full of excitement. He drove with Shelby to the theatre on the back of a monstrous garbage truck they had rented. Quite a few of the hospital staff attended out of courtesy, and for some weeks afterwards Jack, Shelby and Neal found themselves being treated like minor celebrities by the staff, but Jack's dreams for the film died a quick death. The theatre owner wasn't interested in screening the film, and nobody else had seemed to notice.

'The quality might not be the best, but it has an important message,' Jack said.

It was to be a reoccurring theme in Jack's life. The film is an early example of his impulsiveness and the 'do it yourself' methodology that was to be his downfall. He would often develop grand plans, only to be thwarted by his own business naïveté. Inevitably, another exciting idea would come to mind, and the old project would wither.

When the retinal studies had made little impact, he moved on to his plan for death row inmates. When that languished, he decided to create the educational film with Shelby and Neal. With his hopes for the film quickly evaporating, it was only a matter of time before he moved on to another project.

Chapter 6

Blood Brothers

Even though the training film was not the success Jack had hoped for, and even though there would always be those who doubted his research, the staff at Pontiac General supported him, and they were genuinely proud that he had published so many articles at such an early age. He was developing a reputation as a daring researcher, a maverick who, like the great scientific minds of old, would push forward in his quest for truth regardless of the obstacles put in front of him by church, state and the AMA. He was proud of what he had begun to accomplish, and was glad that he could share his successes with his parents.

Although Satenig liked to save the newspaper articles that mentioned Jack's work, she was cautious in her praise of her son. She didn't want him to become conceited, or to get so involved in his work that he lost sight of the many things that make life wonderful. Whenever she saw him she persisted in asking him when he would get married. It was her secret hope that a wife would bring balance into Jack's life, not to mention more grandchildren into hers (she did have one grandchild – Margo's daughter Ava). Her son had always been a bit of an enigma.

Though talkative at home, she always felt that there were aspects of his hopes and fears that he kept hidden from his family. She knew he had always felt a separation from the other kids due to his intelligence, and that as he grew older, though he disguised it well, the feeling of isolation continued. A wife would open him up, give him a best friend he could trust. So when Jack mentioned his work, Satenig always mentioned marriage. Research was something he could always do, but the time for marriage was quickly running out.

Levon liked to needle Jack about marriage as well, but he was quietly confident that his son would get married and settle down as soon as he had established himself as a doctor. What woman could refuse his dashing son's strong, angular features and soulful eyes? His son was a brilliant and handsome man. If he wasn't married, it was only because he hadn't as yet found a woman good enough for him.

Levon loved to ask Jack to tell him about the research he was doing and the many obstacles he faced. He would listen in rapt attention as Jack narrated how his paper presentation in Washington had gone or what the politicians there had said when he was called in to discuss his plan for death row inmates. He felt Jack was speaking one-on-one with the most important people in the nation, and they were listening to him. Although he had nothing but contempt for politicians, due to the Armenian holocaust and the spineless response from America, he felt God saved him from the massacre to beget Jack. He escaped death to sire the death fighter. He felt Jack was destined for greatness and perhaps was in God's great scheme of things to come. Jack was proud of this adulation, this veneration from his beloved father but, as in the past, he was highly embarrassed as well.

Jack felt as content as he ever had in his life. His parents' pride in him bolstered his own pride in the work he did. And he knew, from the way his father's voice had quavered when he called Jack a hero, from the small smile his mother gave him whenever she glanced at him, that what they were really telling him was that they loved him, that they loved the man he had become.

A few weeks after making the training film, a phone call interrupted Jack's hospital rounds. He heard his mother's voice, in between frequent sobs. Something terrible had happened at home.

When Jack first saw his father's body he was surprised at the numbness that took hold of his own, as if he was the one who had suffered a massive heart attack. His father lay there, a cold cadaver like so many others. The doctor in him wanted to be dispassionate; to accept the death as an inevitable and expected end to a full life. But the body in front of him was of his beloved father, not an anonymous collection of tissue and bone. Jack stared, hoping to see Levon miraculously start breathing again. He knew he was being irrational. He had seen death too many times to fall into impractical wishful thinking. Tightness gripped his chest, and no matter how hard he tried he couldn't stop the thoughts and memories that rushed through his mind. In that moment he was no longer Dr Jack Kevorkian, he was only Levon's son Jack, and he had no defence against grief.

In the weeks that followed, he consoled his mother and sisters. Yet Jack himself felt helpless. Doctors for millennia had waged a losing battle against death. They had accomplished so much, extending lifespans and enhancing the quality of life, but for all their efforts they knew so little about their enemy. When death took hold, they fled, leaving the dirty work of dealing with the hereafter to the spiritual community. Jack knew from his research on the history of autopsy that it was possible to strike a blow against death by using the dead to save other's lives. His purpose in life came back into focus. Levon had said that a hero was someone who would take on what others were afraid of. What greater demon was there than death itself, the terror of mankind? Jack felt a new energy welling within. He would find something new, something important to research. It was what his father would have wanted.

Jack turned to the library and read through the medical journals. He quickly became bored with what Western scientists were attempting. Most of their research was similar to what he had encountered among the residents at the University of Michigan: conservative attempts at ameliorating minor problems in a manner likely to offend the least number of people. It disgusted him that the doctors publishing such articles considered themselves researchers.

In one of the journals he came across an article that condemned some Russian research, calling it a violation of human decency. But Jack didn't understand the outrage. According to the article, the Russians were alleviating their blood shortage by taking blood from cadavers for transfusion to patients. Their procedure seemed to work without any ill effects and, most surprisingly, they had apparently been carrying out the procedure for over 40 years.

Jack could barely eat his lunch that day. A nervous excitement filled him. Blood was always in short supply, yet it was essential to the treatment of the critically ill and injured. If they could begin using cadavers, however, the blood shortage would be a distant memory. Jack decided to do his own research to convince himself that cadaver blood transfusions could work. If conducted properly, his research would not only prove that the Russian claims of success were credible, but it would also show which transfusion methods worked better, banked blood or cadaver blood. It wasn't as if this was the first time cadavers had been used to help people survive or have a better quality of life. In the 1880s, a French physician was the first to perform a successful skin transplant from a cadaver to a burn victim. The first kidney transplant from a cadaver, using new tissue-typing techniques and immune suppression drugs, was performed in the US in 1962. By 1967, Dr Christian Barnard was performing the first heart transplant.

But no one in the West, as far as Jack knew, was looking at transfusing blood from a cadaver. Jack wanted to surpass the Russians. He thought it was possible to transfuse blood directly from a corpse into a living human recipient. If he could do that, the process would have potential battlefield benefits. He had seen too many men bleed to death in Korea. It took far too long for medics to transport the wounded to a facility that could transfuse them. Every soldier had their blood type on their dog tags, so a field medic could save countless lives by using the immediately available blood from fallen comrades. He knew the idea might strike some people as macabre, but the benefits far outweighed the squeamishness anyone might have.

In order to properly conduct his work, he would need assistants and volunteers. He immediately turned to Neal and began to explain his ideas. Neal doubted the hospital would approve, but Jack was sure they would. After all, hospital personnel always complained of blood shortages. A cadaver would yield six pints of blood with a 50 per cent higher ratio of red blood cells – and the blood wouldn't require anticoagulants, as blood from live donors would. Why wouldn't they approve? Jack was sure that once he presented all the facts they could get past all the objections from families of the deceased, as well as all the legal hurdles they would face. In order to be sure the process worked, however, he needed human guinea pigs. Neal volunteered to be the first.

Jack camped out in the library to research the cadaver transfusion experiments. If he was going to extend the Russians' research, he had to first understand what, exactly, they had done. Specifics, however, proved difficult to come by. The Russians had first attempted cadaver transfusions in the 1920s because of a shortage of live blood donors. The leader of their efforts was a Dr Shamov, who had first done cadaver transfusions in animals, and then moved on to humans when he perfected his technique. After his first successful case, when he removed blood from the inferior vena cava of a car crash victim and used it to revive a man who had slit his wrists in a suicide attempt, Shamov was encouraged to expand his research. Along with Dr Yudin, who was in charge of the entire surgical and accident department at the Sklifosovsky Institute in Moscow, Shamov performed over 2,500 transfusions in the next few years, and eventually published their results in the renowned medical journal the *Lancet* in 1928.

Their technique wasn't particularly well described, but Jack surmised that the Russian scientists had primarily drawn blood from the cadaver's carotid artery, stored it in a bottle, and then transfused from the bottle to a live patient. Though blood clotted within the cadaver after death, the Russians discovered that enzymes in the blood would naturally dissolve the clots after about an hour. As long as the scientists drained the blood from the cadaver within six hours of death, they found they could salvage 10 to 12 bottles of transfusable blood. They could then flush out the cardiovascular system of the cadaver with a glucose-phosphate solution and obtain a diluted solution of blood products that could be used as a plasma expander. It seemed like a simple procedure, and Jack was confident he could improve on it.

The more he investigated the Russians' techniques, the better the idea seemed to him. One big advantage to using cadaver blood was that a large volume of blood could be obtained from a single cadaver, meaning that a patient who needed a massive transfusion could get all the blood from one source, lessening the chance of a negative reaction to the proteins in the blood from multiple donors. Because of the fibrinolysis effect that broke up the blood clots in the cadaver blood (a process that is to this day not fully understood in medicine) Jack realised that there was no risk of the toxic reactions to anticoagulants that had to be given with live donors. Also, cross matching and testing the blood would be easier, because he would only need to test a sample from the blood donated by the cadaver. Live blood donors could only donate a fraction of what a cadaver could provide, so large blood transfusions were often composed of the blood of several live donors, each of which would need to be tested.

Jack was amazed that a procedure that worked so well had remained relatively unknown. As he looked through his research, however, he found that *The Lancet* had a ready explanation: 'The use of blood from dead bodies seems to be repugnant to the British mind. It has been overcome in Russia, where in this respect, reason triumphed over instinct.' Just as the others had passionately rejected his own retinal experiments and work with death row inmates, ignoring the rationale behind them and instead focusing on how these efforts conflicted with traditional taboos, Jack expected a certain level of resistance to his cadaver transfusion plans. Scientists might eventually grudgingly accept his research, but the general public was always slow to accept change. That was what had happened with his work on death row inmates.

Jack meticulously planned his cadaver blood research so that it was above scientific reproach, he was sure that, in time, other scientists would consider it invaluable. The challenge would be to get the public to agree with them. Jack prepared his proposal and took it to the hospital administrators. He first stopped by the office of John Marra, the head of pathology for the hospital at the time. Jack expected Dr Marra to have doubts, but he hoped that if he explained his proposal thoroughly Dr Marra would recognise the benefits and grudgingly allow Jack to test the proposal out a few times. While Dr Marra listened, Jack went through the key points, emphasising that the procedure would save lives, that it was clearly safe because the Russians had already tested it thousands of times, and that, even if the public reacted when they found out what research had been going on at the hospital, that at least the military would back them because of the obvious favourable battlefield applications. The longer he spoke, though, the more nervous Jack became, and he was surprised when Dr Marra agreed to take his proposal to the hospital administrators.

When Jack was called in to talk to the administrators a few days later, the meeting felt like a celebration in his honour. The administrators shook his hand, all of them smiling, eager to hear more details about his proposal. They even told Jack that some of the staff had already asked if they could work with him on this research.

Jack soon found that in addition to Neal Nicol's assistance, he now had offers of help from Dr Marra, Dr Glenn Byslma and others. This support fuelled Jack's confidence. These doctors respected him and believed in him nearly as much as his father had. Instead of feeling like a pariah engaged in a solitary crusade, he felt like a respected researcher whose work would be taken seriously. He realised, though, that in order for that respect to continue, his proposal would have to succeed. He would have to do more than just duplicate and verify the Russian claims of success with cadaver blood transfusions; he would have to improve on what they had done.

With some trepidation, Jack and Neal began what Jack would later call 'my first real extraction of human benefit from death'. It wasn't hard to get the cadaver blood; the hospital had a plentiful supply of patients who had recently died from heart attacks, strokes or accidents. After they gained consent from relatives to use their loved one's bodies for these experiments, they would perform a quick autopsy, put the cadaver on a tilt table, insert a tube into the jugular and let the blood drain into a bottle. When they transfused the blood into volunteers, they found surprisingly few side effects. Two of the first four reported no problems, while the other two reported only mild discomfort at the injection site. This effect is also exhibited with banked blood. Temperature variations from refrigerator to live recipients, dissatisfaction with the venipuncture and a concern about getting a transfusion can all stimulate such discomfort. Jack, in collaboration with Glenn Bylsma, published the results in the May 1961 issue of the *American Journal of Clinical Pathology*.

In the article, Jack acknowledged that some would consider the experiment only a partial success since two of the four patients had experienced side effects. Rather than focus on how minor these 'failures' were, however, Jack focused on the benefits of the procedure. He wrote, 'The blood is free – requiring no remuneration either on the part of the hospital or the coroner … cadaver blood is ideal … for indigent patients.' Not only would the process save money, but also 'routine consent from the recipient is no more necessary than in instances of conventional bank blood transfusions'.

More experiments were conducted on patients at the hospital. Consent was obtained from the deceased's next of kin to perform an autopsy, which allowed the blood to be taken. Any patients who were transfused with cadaver blood were informed of its source and allowed to choose either cadaver or bank blood. Most of these patients were elderly, suffering from severe anaemia or leukaemia, where the haemoglobin was dangerously low and patients would have required multiple transfusions from many sources. Their participation was strictly voluntary.

When people needed blood, it didn't really matter where it came from so long as it saved their lives. Since cadavers were a perfect source of free blood, it simply made sense to make use of them. Once again, Jack relied on the readers of his article to look at the situation rationally. For those who might argue that the procedure violated the sanctity of the body, or who raised religious arguments centred on the line between life and death, Jack was blunt. He wrote, 'Most of these objections are more imaginary than real.' It wasn't that he was unwilling to deal with the objections; he merely thought that they were inconsequential in the face of the staggering benefits the cadaver blood transfusion procedure promised.

Jack expected his article to generate debate. He welcomed it. The benefits of cadaver blood transfusions were clear, and with time, the process could be honed to perfection. If there was an objection, he didn't expect it to last long. It would be a while before enough people read the article, in any case. the *American Journal of Clinical Pathology* was a fine publication, but it definitely wasn't a bestseller.

To his surprise, members of the hospital staff greeted him at the end of May with a *Time* magazine article that mentioned his work. Within weeks of the publication of his results, his research had become national news again. But once again it was for the wrong reasons. Rather than focus on the extensive benefits of the procedure that he'd listed in his article, the *Time* article expressed its horror at 'the case of a 49-year-old woman in the Pontiac General Hospital who was given two pints of blood from the cadaver of a 12-year-old boy who had drowned in a nearby lake and who had been dead for two-and-a-half to three hours'. The crime, apparently, had been in using the blood of a drowned boy. Jack was furious. It had seemed to him that he had found a way to preserve a spark of life in the wake of a senseless death, that what he had done had been a beautiful way to honour and respect the young boy, but the article made him seem like a mad scientist obsessed with the macabre. Statements from his article were quoted out of context and listed as further evidence of the bizarre nature of his work. Jack was incredulous. It was as if the writer of the article had consciously gone out of his way to present Jack in the worst light.

Although the staff had accepted Jack when he first entered the hospital, the *Time* article revealed that acceptance only went so far. As Michael Betzold reported in his book *Appointment with Doctor Death*:

> Dr Murray Levin, then an internist at Pontiac General, said Kevorkian's frequent talk about his research unnerved his colleagues.

'Most of us just sort of changed the subject when he got on it,' Levin said. 'We thought it was inappropriate. We had plenty of blood. We didn't need to deal with cadavers.'

Though the hospital, in actuality, didn't have 'plenty of blood', Dr Levin's comments represented a common perception among the staff who were now becoming leery of Jack's work. For them, the hospital had been doing well enough with the blood supply it had. Tapping into cadavers to augment that supply simply wasn't worth the trade-off. Sure, cadaver blood was less expensive and much easier to transfuse, but if they worked with it they opened themselves up to the same condemnations that had been levelled at Jack. The best career move was to distance themselves from Jack, at least until his work had been accepted.

Once again, Jack was more surprised to find that he still had some supporters at the hospital, including Dr Marra, Dr Bylsma and Neal Nicol. They had worked closely with Jack and had seen the effect of the cadaver transfusions. With Jack's persistent optimism about how the procedure would revolutionise transfusions, it was difficult for them to cultivate doubt. They believed in him nearly as much as he believed in himself, and with such a strong cadre supporting him, Jack felt he couldn't fail.

Next, he wanted to go beyond what the Russians had done. They had used a two-step process, where the blood went from the cadaver to a bottle, and from the bottle to a patient. Jack saw a practical application – on the battlefield – for a one-step process, straight from the cadaver to the patient. Once again, however, he would need human guinea pigs to test his theory.

Though Jack's confidence, and to some extent his notoriety, persuaded a number of people to volunteer, Neal Nicol pushed to be the first test subject during the clinical research on direct transfusion of cadaver blood. He had been with Jack before the press had become interested in the transfusion research and the two had long before discussed the possibility of direct transfusion. He understood that there were risks involved with being a test subject, but he was certain nothing unexpected would transpire as long as he was in Jack's hands.

One day the perfect cadaver for Jack's research turned up at the hospital. The donor was a 30-year-old man who had died unexpectedly from a massive heart attack, but who was otherwise healthy. They had been looking for a younger donor whose condition was similar to that of a typical battlefield victim, and for all intents and purposes they had found one. Though a heart attack victim dies in shocking quiet, as if a switch has suddenly gone off inside them, their physical condition, as far as transfusion is concerned, is no different from what one would find in a soldier with a gunshot wound to the head.

The cadaver had been dead for less than six hours when he was wheeled in. Jack and Neal were both nervously excited. The two quickly drew a few vials of blood from the cadaver and performed a series of compatibility tests. The cadaver's blood type was O positive, and since Jack's blood type meant that he could only receive AB positive, Neal was a perfect candidate for the cadaver blood. Jack quickly removed a pint of Neal's blood so that his circulatory system wouldn't be overloaded when the cadaver blood was transfused into him. Both understood the importance of the moment, they had both been stationed overseas and had heard too many horror stories about men in battle bleeding to death because of a lack of easily transfusable blood.

Jack asked Neal if he still wanted to go through with it. Neal answered, 'Hell, yes.' The two lingered a bit, easing their nervousness with banter, until finally Neal lay down on the floor beside the tilt table the cadaver was on. Jack inserted a syringe pump into the jugular of the cadaver, then ran a line from the pump to Neal's arm. In the next 30 minutes, Neal received 400cc of blood, experiencing only a slight coolness at the injection site. When they were done Neal sat up almost immediately, and the two began the necessary post-transfusion studies.

Their next transfusion, on another male volunteer, went as smoothly as the one with Neal. The procedure was simple and nearly fail-proof – even an untrained soldier could probably do it. The results excited Jack so much that he was certain the military would be banging on his door as soon as he published the research. With their backing and financial support he could make cadaver blood transfusions as common as vaccines.

Jack wanted to do one more test before he began publishing his results, and for this one he wanted a female test subject. Some of the female staff had volunteered long before his first test on Neal, and with rumours floating around the hospital about how successful the last two tests had been Jack had no problem finding a volunteer to receive the transfusion. When the partially mangled body of a 14-year-old hit-and-run victim was wheeled in, Jack finally had his donor. But while he and Neal were busy testing the girl's blood, the volunteer stood in shock beside the body.

Jack told her that she had an opportunity to do something good from a senseless tragedy. The volunteer lay down and closed her eyes.

They spent the next few minutes in silence, the volunteer lying quietly, Jack and Neal busy double-checking the compatibility tests. When they were finally ready, Jack attached an intravenous line to the volunteer while Neal prepped the cadaver.

There was a problem, Neal said. They couldn't go through the jugular.

Jack stood up and walked over to the cadaver. Neal was right. The horrific injuries the girl had sustained on the rest of her body paled in comparison with what had happened to her neck. Abraded and crushed by the hit-and-run driver's car, there was little to distinguish between skin, bone and cartilage. Even if they could find the girl's jugular, there was no guarantee it could withstand the pressures of the transfusion.

Jack knew he had to find a way to make it work. A medic in the field would see worse injuries than that. If this procedure was going to be of interest to the military, it had to be applicable even when the medic couldn't easily reach the jugular. He snatched the syringe pump out of Neal's hands and plunged it into the cadaver's heart. Blood immediately began to course through the line to the volunteer's body.

Neal stood in shock. He knew that the public would also be shocked.

The volunteer interrupted them with a low moan. When Neal asked what was wrong, she said that she had a bitter taste in her mouth. Jack exchanged a worried look with Neal. They had never heard anything remotely similar during the other occasions. Jack bent down and took the volunteer's pulse. It was strong, her breathing steady.

The volunteer struggled to get up, and her eyes were glazed.

Immediately telling her to lie back down, Jack turned to Neal to make sure they had screened the blood. They had. Jack got up and pulled the syringe pump from the cadaver's heart. Neal

quickly disconnected the tubing from the volunteer. She stag-
gered to her feet and stumbled towards the chair where she'd left
her purse, assuring the men that she felt perfectly fine.

Neal asked Jack what they should do. Jack's advice was to keep
an eye on her while they retested the blood, and to take her to
the ER if she got any worse. Jack wheeled the cadaver out of the
room. Neal spent the next hour with the volunteer, giving her
water, talking to her. Slowly she became less disoriented, until
finally she was able to walk out of the room on her own.

When Neal later ran into Jack, Jack greeted him with a smile.
Neal was anxious to find out what Jack had discovered – and
was shocked to learn that the volunteer was 'just drunk'. Neal
expressed disbelief that she'd come in for a research experiment
in that condition. Jack said she hadn't – it turned out that the
deceased had been drunk when she was hit by the car, and the
volunteer had been feeling the effects of the alcohol the victim
had consumed.

Jack spent the next few weeks preparing an article on their research.
Although the transfusion procedure could be used by anyone, he
focused on the military application. If he simply reported the results
of his trials he was sure his work would be dismissed again, but by
including the military application of the procedure he hoped his
work would find easier acceptance. The new technique would dramatically increase the accessibility of transfusions on the battlefield,
and reduce the delay before they could be administered. He again
listed the benefits of using cadaver blood over live donor blood and
prepared a description of the equipment medical corpsmen would
need in order to perform the procedure.

By the time he was done, he had written a clear explanation

of the transfusion procedure and how it could immediately be implemented in the military. The military, he believed, wouldn't allow itself to be held hostage by religious objections because the war in Vietnam was reaching its crescendo. He was sure they were an audience that would see the merits of his work and put the procedure into practice, thus easing the way for a wider public acceptance of his methods.

Jack submitted the article to the Pentagon with a grant proposal. He offered to conduct continuing research with Neal, if necessary in the battlefield conditions of Vietnam. After a few months he received a curt response from the military, similar to the response he was getting from other scientists who had read his article. The procedure looked promising, but needed further evaluation. His doubters questioned his research, saying that he still needed to perform tests to see if cadaver blood had the same viability as live donor blood. As well, he needed to prove that the cadaver blood wouldn't cause some unforeseen side effect down the line. Typically, Jack was annoyed at the suggestions. He thought questioning the long-term safety of cadaver blood was as irrelevant as questioning whether it was better to drink a soda out of a can or a bottle.

However as the military did seem interested, Jack was willing to do a little bit more research to prove that the procedure was safe. First, he honed the extraction technique to maximise the red cell content of the cadaver blood, building on ideas that had come up during the initial rounds of cadaver transfusion. Once that was in hand, he began preparation for a comparison test between cadaver blood and live donor blood from the blood bank. He quickly realised that the best way to measure cell survival time in the blood was by tagging the cells with a slightly radioactive isotope. The isotope wouldn't affect how the blood performed, nor would its radioactivity pose any health threats, but by measuring how slowly the radioactivity decayed in the different samples, Jack could determine how long the blood was maintaining its cellular integrity. After the initial tests showed that blood left in bottles degraded at an equal rate in both live and cadaver blood, Jack prepared to perform similar tests on blood transfused into volunteers.

Jack, Neal and one of their diehard volunteers, a lab technician name Bill Beaubien, acted as the control group, using blood from the blood bank. Jack excitedly began preparing the article and a separate synopsis for the military. A few weeks later, Neal had some troubling news. Both he and Bill were feeling ill. Jack realised that he too had been feeling under the weather. He looked closer at Neal. Neal's eyes had an orange tint, and his skin bore the telltale yellow of jaundice. Jack suggested that because they had all used the same blood from the blood bank, they should all get tested for hepatitis.

The irony of the situation immediately struck home. In the next months, those volunteers who had received cadaver blood continued on as if nothing had happened. The three who had received blood from the supposedly safe blood bank, however, all contracted hepatitis. Jack and Bill suffered the least, working through their sickness, but Neal was incapacitated for six months.

It seemed like they had definitive proof that cadaver blood transfusions were as safe, if not safer, than live donor transfusions. The research was eventually published in the *Journal of Military Medicine* in January 1964, but the military passed on Jack's proposal without comment. Jack was furious. He resolved 'never again to waste time and effort in futile appeals for support from government agencies'.

He would find a way to go it completely alone if that's what it took to do real research.

Jack gave up his work on cadaver transfusions. Neither the military – nor anyone else – has ever perfected or used the technique in any practical application. Although methods of testing banked blood for diseases such as hepatitis and AIDS (unknown at the time Jack was testing his transfusions) have much improved, the transfusion process has changed very little.

Still reeling from the military's rejection of the cadaver blood transfusion studies, Jack received a call from his sisters. Satenig had abdominal cancer, and there wasn't much the doctors could do for her. Jack refused to believe it and decided to look over the hospital records for himself. He tracked down the cancer specialists and asked their opinion, but they just repeated what the other doctors had already said. It was nearly impossible to surgically remove all the tumours that pervaded her abdomen, and if they tried she might die on the operating table. Chemotherapy was an option, but the drugs they had available weren't very effective.

Jack frequently visited his mother in hospital, but he was helpless to do anything other than hold her hand and tell her he loved her. The doctors in charge of her care fought to keep her alive, ordering endless blood tests so they could pump her body with the highest level of chemotherapy she could handle. At first Satenig winced at the needle pricks, but as the months wore on she barely moved when the nurses came with their syringes, even when the trainee nurses sometimes jabbed their needle past the vein and into a muscle.

Jack was beside himself with worry and chided the nurses for incompetence. They, in trepidation of the doctor, tried to explain that his mother didn't have a lot of good veins they could work with. Satenig, in turn, reprimanded her son for being insensitive to the nurses, saying she couldn't feel the needle anyway because of the general excruciating pain she was enduring.

As the doctors' tests would later reveal, the cancer had spread into Satenig's bones; she had no chance of recovering.

Jack tried to get the doctors to increase the amount of morphine his mother was receiving to control the pain, but the doctors politely refused. Jack argued that the morphine might relieve her pain, and certainly wouldn't hurt her. But the doctors still refused. If they upped the dose, they said, she would be comatose most of the time – and probably get addicted to the morphine as well.

'Addiction isn't something she has to worry about. It's the pain! The best you can do is make sure she doesn't feel any pain!' Jack yelled.

But the doctors were steadfast. Giving Satenig more morphine had the potential to do her harm, and so they couldn't risk it. They felt the Hippocratic oath was clear on that point. Jack could only shake his head and walk away. There was no use yelling at the doctors, they were following standard hospital procedure. As Jack went through the rest of his day, he was surprised to find his hands shaking at the most inopportune times. It was as if his body wanted him to do something, anything, if it meant his mother might feel less pain, but his body was being held in check by his mind, by the part of him that knew the way hospitals worked. The doctors would never admit that the cancer had won and that the best thing they could do was try to give his mother as much comfort and as painless a death as possible. In their eyes she wasn't a woman facing an agonising death, but solely a reminder of their latest battle in the war against cancer.

Jack watched his mother die in pain, helpless to do anything to help her. During the days he wasn't with her Jack buried himself in his work, hoping that nestled amidst the cold facts and procedures of a pathology lab he might get some peace. But the pathology lab did little to help. The peaceful dead, bodies that felt nothing when sliced with a scalpel, surrounded him. He kept thinking of how his mother continued to suffer, how the doctors would fight relentlessly to give her another day of life, even if that day was nothing more than another day of torture. It was as if she had never escaped the Turks in Armenia, as if, somehow, the nightmares of her past had somehow found a way to torment her in the present, luring Jack's medical peers into the role of torturers.

Though Jack didn't know it, his sisters secretly begged the doctors to end their mother's life, but the doctors refused. Satenig lingered on for several more months, delirious from the pain. When she died, Jack and his sisters quietly held a small ceremony. Though filled with sadness, they also felt a sense of relief. Their mother was at last at peace.

Chapter 7

The Wilderness Years

The sense of relief that Jack felt at his mother's funeral was short lived, and soon he found himself questioning both himself and the medical profession. Doctors were well trained to deal with most situations, but when faced with the inevitability of a painful death they generally attempted to avoid the issue. When pain continued after prescribed medicine failed to help, they felt inadequate and resorted to equivocation and prevarication. They were poor pain managers.

There wasn't anything wrong with a doctor tenaciously fighting to preserve life, but Jack was astonished that no one seemed to consider the possibility that surrender was sometimes the best option. They faced death every day, and yet they tried to ignore its power, or its natural role in life as a necessary and inevitable end. Although he had not yet begun thinking in terms of assisted suicide, in his research Jack had tried to map the boundaries of death, to find ways to reap some benefit for the living, and he was sure he had much to say on the topic that the medical community needed to hear. But no one seemed to want to listen.

Instead, Jack began to try to communicate through art. He had always enjoyed drawing cartoons or doodling, and when he had been the cartoonist for the high-school paper he'd found that the forum was a convenient way to communicate a message to a large group of people. He enrolled in an evening adult education oil painting class at a nearby school, but was annoyed when he discovered that the other students were only interested in duplicating pictures of clowns, flowers and landscapes. Jack combined his understanding of the human anatomy with his fascination with death and created works that author Michael Betzold described in his book *Appointment with Doctor Death* as '... bold and strident, as critical and unforgiving, as pointed and dramatic as Kevorkian's own fighting words. They are strikingly well-executed, stark and surreal – and frightening, demented and /or hilarious, depending on one's point of view.' If all the other students were interested in painting clichés, Jack decided he would try to create something so weird it would shock them speechless.

Most of his paintings depicted war and death. His experience working with cadavers, some delivered after gruesome accidents, gave his depictions of amputated limbs and decapitated heads an almost photographic realism. Jack wielded his images as symbols, relentlessly driving a message home with his work. In the painting *Nearer My God to Thee* a screaming body falls down a pit towards a black abyss populated with ghostly faces, futilely trying to grasp on to the walls with fingers that have been worn to bone. For him, death brought only nothingness. Jack wrote descriptions to go along with each of his paintings when they were exhibited in Michigan in 1994. He said of *Nearer My God to Thee*:

Despite the solace of specious religiosity and its seductive prom-
ise of an after-life of heavenly bliss, most of us will do anything
to thwart the inevitable victory of biological death. We contem-
plate and face it with great apprehension, profound fear, and
paralyzing terror, sparing no financial or physical sacrifice, pleading wantonly and unashamedly, clutching any hope of salvation
through medicine or prayer. How forbidding that dark abyss.
How stupendous the yearning to dodge its gaping orifice. How
inevitable the engulfment. Yet, below are the disintegrating hulks
of those who have gone before; they have made the insensible
transition and wonder what the fuss is all about. After all, how
excruciating can nothingness be?'

Jack's depiction of death itself was a haunting signal of what he
was feeling so soon after the deaths of his parents. In a later 1991
interview with the *Detroit Free Press*, Jack said dreams about his
parents still woke him up at night and made him wonder about
death. He explained, 'if you don't have any sort of faith, you think
of the big nothingness, and you wonder, "What is this brief span of
consciousness?" "What is all this?" All thinking people go through
this – you just don't talk about it. There's no answer, anyway.' In
these days of raw grief, instead of talking he painted.

Although Jack had allowed himself to relax and make friends
while at Pontiac General, his reaction to his parents' death was to
draw in on himself. He maintained that pure unreasoned emotion led to trouble. Though the outside world might not mind
riding an emotional roller coaster, Jack wanted to live his life
with more intellectual restraint, and he tried to ensure that his
friends did so as well.

For instance, when John F Kennedy was assassinated, Jack noticed how quickly the nation abandoned reason in favour of emotion. Although the conspiracy theories would come in time, Jack found that the lunchroom discussions were already hot and heated in the days after Kennedy's death. With little to go on other than news footage of the assassination itself, most of the people that Jack encountered believed that the only accept-able thing to do was to exact an equal measure of revenge on Kennedy's assassin.

When Jack sat down at the lunch table, he saw that Neal had everyone's attention. Neal wanted to make an example of Lee Harvey Oswald; he thought he should be castrated and then hung. Jack, on the other hand, felt that Oswald should be treated no differently than any other murderer – no matter who it was he had killed.

Jack had made his point. If society did treat Oswald differently, it would be making the mistake of allowing emotion and irrationality govern its actions and, as Jack was eager to point out, emotion and irrationality were at the root of mankind's biggest debacles, from rejection of scientific innovations to the scarring of genocide and wars. If there were to be any hope for mankind, its people would have to get past emotional knee-jerk responses, and instead actively try to live up to a higher principled standard that was applied to everyone equally. True justice, and true equality, required it.

A female colleague of Jack's was aked to leave the hospital when they found out she was pregnant. Unmarried, she found her-self with no means to support herself or her child. Jack thought this entirely unfair. Again, it was an example of society's irration-ality. He found himself thinking about the societal reaction to pregnancy, how women were the ones who always bore the brunt of the responsibility and were the ones whose lives were most dramatically affected. It ultimately didn't matter if the woman was married or not, she was expected to sacrifice everything in order to raise the child. It would be better if both men and women were capable of bearing children, Jack thought, because then at least society would be forced to acknowledge the extent of the sacrifice required to bear a child.

Jack mentioned to Neal an article about in vitro fertilisation research being conducted in Italy. The attempt to nurture a foetus outside the constraints of the womb seemed like a promising field of science, and one which might make it possible for both men and women to bear children. It seemed amazing to him that such research was going on in Italy, despite the stranglehold on science that the Roman Catholic Church held there, but it was clear that the research needed a lot more work if it was going to succeed. The Italian researcher, Petruchi, could only sustain life in the fertilised eggs for a short time because the Petri dish in which the embryos were stored did a poor job of imitating the womb. The researcher had been meticulously introducing nutrients into the Petri dishes and trying to remove the wastes that built up, but his technique was a poor substitute for the circulatory system in the womb that easily removed toxic wastes and replenished the embryo's nutritional needs.

Neal jokingly suggested there might be a way to implant a fertilised egg in a man's belly. This had already occurred to Jack, who noted that in the abdominal cavity, which is rich in blood vessels, one might be able to create an environment that would mimic the womb. Once again, Neal volunteered his services as guinea pig number one.

Despite their optimism, they found no support from the few hospital staff they spoke to about it. Their plan to implant an embryo in Neal died quickly when their efforts to find a research facility that would help them turned up few promising leads. The facilities were either apprehensive of having Jack Kevorkian performing research in their labs, or of having such controversial research going on in their buildings. Still, the two persisted in their search, looking for ways to get funding. They didn't need much, they were willing to work without pay, but the equipment they required would either have to be borrowed or paid for at great expense. Jack eventually established Penumbra, Inc as the name of their research organisation. He hoped that by using the name 'Penumbra', which means the time between dark and dawn and symbolises an awakening, he could better attract funds than if he used his own name. It didn't matter though. No one was interested in supporting their research. The only positive outcome was that Jack could use Penumbra to seek funding for his work in the future, but that provided little solace at the time.

In fact, Jack and Neal's difficulties in trying to get their research supported represented only a hint of the difficulties Jack was to face in the years to come. Just as the Italian researcher who had conducted the in vitro fertilisation studies had suddenly seen his funding disappear when the Catholic Church found out what he was up to, Jack and Neal found that they had very few backers who were willing to support any research that could potentially offend the church of the common public. With limited funds at their disposal, and nearly no support for the research they had done in the past, it seemed like their adventures were nearing an end.

When Jack's proponent and friend Dr Marra retired, Jack assumed the position of Chief Pathologist. Jack did not, nor does not, suffer fools gladly and he deemed one of his assistants just that. He took little time in dismissing him by having his desk removed from his office and placed in the hall (so much for the rational, reasoned responses he espoused). The administration disagreed with Jack's precipitous decision and during the ensuing argument Jack quit the position and the hospital.

For a man unaccustomed to compromise the decision was easy. Jack left the hospital, confident that the doctor shortage would mean that another hospital would hire him on the spot. Neal had already left to take a job in laboratory sales, and though he still kept in touch with Jack, the heady days when they could research anything seemed over. Neal had to focus on his work and his career. It would keep him anchored in Michigan, and eventually cause him to lose touch with Jack.

Jack found it much more difficult to find employment. When he followed the traditional route of submitting his résumé, none of the hospitals called him in for an interview. 'My curriculum vitae scares the hell out of people,' he said. He soon discovered that it was easier to walk into a hospital, talk to the chief pathologist, and then offer to fill in when the pathologist was on vacation. It worked every time. The lab personnel and hospital staff were often so pleased with his performance that they would plead with the chief pathologist when he returned from vacation to hire Jack. Only when Jack joined the staff would he be required to submit his résumé, and by that time the hospital wouldn't care; they had found a competent pathologist and didn't mind his chequered history.

In this way Jack was able to pick up a job as an associate pathologist at Wyandotte General Hospital, but the work soon bored him and he chaffed under the rigid administration of the hospital, so after 18 months he left to pursue an independent venture. He opened the Checkup Diagnostic Center, a 'multiphase diagnostic clinic' set up to provide preventative care by enabling walk-in clients to receive an analysis of their health status based on a battery of lab tests and X-rays. The Center gave Jack a chance to be his own boss, and he enjoyed the freedom this gave him. Also, he enjoyed helping clients determine how best to handle their health conditions, and took particular joy in helping them understand the meaning behind all the lab results.

Most walk-in clients entered with the same level of fear and trepidation that patients at a hospital would – in the late 1960s medical science was an unknown, and often scary, field that seemed to require unending blood draws and large, pulsating machines. Jack took great pride in putting his clients at their ease. He would sit down with them and explain everything at length, and the patients left feeling that they finally understood what was going on with them. Most doctors would tell the patient what was wrong and what they planned to do, but they rarely explained how the treatment they proposed was linked to the ailment being treated. Jack took his time to explain – that was what the clinic was all about. He was certain that as more patients referred him to others, and as doctors began to refer more patients to him, the business would slowly, but steadily grow until he had a business with enough cash flow to fund his research.

Unfortunately, the clinic only lasted a year and a half. Though based on a good idea, the venture failed because it couldn't generate enough business. Jack would later bitterly claim that the failure was because 'other doctors felt competition and were frightened' but the truth was that Jack's inexperience as a businessman doomed the business from the start. Reluctant to put money into advertising the business, and reliant on patient referrals and referrals from doctors to fuel his patient base, Jack simply couldn't draw enough clients to turn a profit. His expectation that other doctors would refer their patients to him was a case of wishful thinking. Although many doctors respected his clinic and felt that it provided competent analysis of lab and X-ray results, they were expected to refer patients who needed diagnostic tests to the appropriate labs within their own hospital; that was, after all, an important income for hospitals. When the lab experienced financial problems it was purchased by another Armenian and became one of the largest reference laboratories in the state, undertaking sophisticated procedures doctors and hospitals lacked the proper equipment to do.

Though disillusioned with the medical profession, Jack again tried to find employment in a hospital, and was pleasantly surprised when he was picked as the chief pathologist at Detroit's Saratoga General Hospital in 1970. Jack dived into the work at the hospital and initially enjoyed his duties there. But again, the longer he worked the more disinterested he became in the routine of the hospital. His time was taken up by administrative duties and his responsibilities in the pathology department; he had little time to devote to research. It frustrated him that his life had devolved into such a routine. The job might have been considered the pinnacle of another doctor's career, but for Jack it just didn't feel like enough.

However, it was while at Saratoga General that Jack had his most serious romantic relationship. The regular hours at the hospital freed time for Jack, and he began dating. Most of the women he encountered didn't live up to his standards, and after a brief dinner or a movie, he would move on. But one woman was different. Her name was Jane, and she was a clerk at a store Jack frequented. Although she knew little of medicine and worked as a store clerk, Jack found that he could talk to her honestly. He didn't feel awkward in her presence and enjoyed meeting with her, especially after a long day spent drudging through administrative work at the hospital. Young and beautiful, intelligent and warm, she seemed to be everything that he could hope for. Recalling his parents' desires for him to get married, Jack finally got up the nerve to ask the woman if she would marry him.

Their engagement was short lived. Although Jane seemed deeply in love with Jack, he began to grow disenchanted. She had come from a good family and should have completed her education, but she had dropped out of a ritzy private college after one semester. That to Jack seemed like evidence that she was undisciplined and didn't have ambition. When he began to goad her about her goals, her dreams, she would talk about marriage and children.

After a few months of his questions Jane withdrew into herself and became more sullen. The final straw was when Jack took her to a park to listen to classical German music. She had asked him to take her out someplace interesting, but now that he had, she was petulant.

Jack didn't understand. She'd said she wanted to have fun, hadn't she? This was music that Jack liked, and he presumed she would enjoy it too. He had never asked her what she would like to do, and when she expressed this to Jack, he felt she was wasting her time by being unhappy about the situation.

After Jack dropped her off at her home that night, he broke off the engagement and never contacted her again. He later ruminated that his rejection of marriage was the biggest mistake of his life. He could have had companionship and children. His failure to do so meant that he was 'shirking responsibility as a human being'. From nature's standpoint, he felt himself dissolute.

Soon after he ended his engagement, in 1976, he quit his job at Saratoga General. Disillusioned by medicine, and disillusioned by the thought of marriage, he wanted to find something creative to do with his life. It occurred to him that he could combine his love of art and music by making a movie of one of his favourite compositions: Handel's *Messiah*. He wasn't particularly interested in movies, and he wasn't exactly sure how to go about creating a feature length film, but June 23rd, 1976, Jack packed up all his belongings into his beige 1968 Volkswagen van and set off for California.

A pork pie hat squashed low on his forehead, his body hunched over the wheel, his only thoughts were on the road ahead and the movie he planned to make. He didn't think there was anything left for him in Michigan except his friendship with Neal and the memories of a childhood spent in the home his father had built in Pontiac. He believed his medical career was essentially over. He could still try to advance his research, but few journals were willing to publish his controversial work, and even fewer hospitals were willing to have him on their staff. He thought he knew he could continue to get part-time positions at hospitals as long as the doctor shortage made them willing to hire qualified professionals without asking for a résumé, but the doctor shortage wouldn't last forever. At the age of 48, with few real prospects for his medical career, he was eager to explore the other paths in life.

Jack was certain that he could make a full-length feature film that would open up new opportunities for him. With his penny-pinching savvy, he naïvely thought it wouldn't be too difficult to make a good film in Hollywood using his life savings as the budget. He felt he had learned a lot about handling a camera from his experiences creating the training film at Pontiac General, and he had a great movie idea he believed would have universal appeal. He thought a movie based on Handel's *Messiah* couldn't fail with him directing it; people would fill theatres just to hear the music alone.

The *Messiah* had captivated Jack ever since he first heard it as a child. Separated in three parts, the *Messiah* represents Christ's birth, death and resurrection through a series of arias and choruses based on biblical passages. What most inspired Jack was Christ's perseverance in the face of martyrdom. Listening to the music when a journal rejected his research or a hospital didn't hire him helped keep things in perspective. Reinterpreting the *Messiah* through film seemed the most logical way to pay homage.

Jack wanted to reinvent the *Messiah* in a way that would appeal to an even larger audience than the piece had enjoyed during its Victorian era heyday. Back then, the push to bring music to the common man as a way of instilling a sense of morality had led to huge festivals at Crystal Palace that routinely used over 3,000 performers to entertain tens of thousands. Those performances caused a radical shift in the way music was viewed in England; it was no longer solely the domain of the wealthy, but had instead become integrated in the lives of people of all classes. Jack felt that in the 20th century classical music had lost appeal to the common man and was quickly becoming something to which only the intellectual elite paid attention. A movie would reach far more people than the Crystal Palace performances had, and in a more visceral way.

As Jack considered how he could stretch his life savings so that it covered the costs of renting equipment for the movie and hiring the actors, he felt an excitement that had been missing from his life ever since the cadaver blood transfusions with Neal Nicol. He hoped that his *Messiah* would do as much for him as the original had for Handel. Handel had created one of the most renowned pieces of English music, a work so magical that he would be forever remembered as one of the great classical composers. For Jack, whose best efforts as a researcher were largely ignored, creating a film of Handel's *Messiah* carried the possibility of redemption.

Jack was too busy during his first weeks in Los Angeles to find an apartment he could afford, so he slept in his van. It didn't bother him. Jack thought that making the film would be fairly easy, that as long as he was near Hollywood, he would be able to find the necessary cameras and actors. He drove his van to film studio lots and asked to borrow equipment, and when he saw someone that he could use in his movie, he asked if they wanted to accept the part. He explained that he was going to make a movie of the *Messiah*, and that it would be something fresh and new. Not a typical Hollywood movie, but one with class and real intrinsic value. When people asked him if he had directed or written a movie before, he mentioned the training film, explaining that there really wasn't any difference between what he had done in Michigan and what he planned on doing in Los Angeles. The *Messiah* film might be a bigger project, but Handel had already written the screenplay and, as far as Jack was concerned, all a director needed was a clear vision for the film and the ability to focus a camera. He couldn't understand why everyone seemed to question the legitimacy of what he was doing, or his ability to pull it off. He had the willingness, the time and he thought the money to create the film, and that was all that should matter.

But to those Jack talked to near the studio lots, he seemed deluded. Men wearing Salvation Army clothes and a pork pie hat didn't make real movies. Major studios, like MGM and FOX, controlled the movies; Jack was again trying to go against the established routes, two decades before the transition to independent producers occurred.

Jack didn't have any success snaring professional actors, but Los Angeles was filled with aspiring stars. He discovered that if he took the time to explain his plan to these young actors, his own excitement often persuaded them. He soon had a band of eager hopefuls ready to create the film with him. The only problem was that none had any real training. Jack hoped their enthusiasm would make up for this loss.

Jack next set out to rent a 35mm motion picture camera. The rental price of a camera, though, was much steeper than Jack had anticipated. The movie was going to cost far more than he'd expected, but he was sure he'd make the money back once the movie was shown.

One of the men who offered to rent Jack equipment also gave him a tip of the trade. One way to cut costs was to use stock footage. Film studios had storage rooms filled with reels of footage that hadn't been used in other films and could be purchased on the cheap. Jack began making the rounds of the studios, his script in hand, looking for footage that would fit his film. Though he was able to pick up a lot of material cheaply, the footage wasn't of great quality or particularly relevant. Jack was in a bind. He didn't have the budget to film the movie the way he wanted it, so he was forced to make compromises. He hoped that if the audience was overwhelmed by Handel's music, the poor quality of the visual wouldn't bother them. The music would capture their imagination, and the images on the screen would become a visual melody, more metaphor than narrative.

Using the music of the *Messiah* as his guide, Jack composed the screenplay. Since he couldn't afford the necessary audio equipment to capture actors' dialogue, he was forced to revert back to the days of silent movies and dub in the music on the soundtrack. He used magnificent recordings from the University of Michigan Choral Union and the Interlochen Arts Academy Orchestra. He shot a series of small biblical scenes with actors, which he intended to intersperse with the stock footage as if they were instruments in the orchestra, flashing visual notes on the screen in tune with the ebb and flow of the music.

There is only eighteen minutes left of Jack's movie, *An Abridged Screen Adaptation of the Oratorio* Messiah *by George Frederic Handel,* because all the film canisters were accidentally lost by the California warehouse in which they had been stored. The entire film was made up of poorly re-enacted biblical scenes, stock footage and surrealistic images whose meanings were clear to Jack, but no one else. For instance, when the music moves into the mezzo-soprano Recitatif 'Behold, a virgin shall conceive', the audience sees a woman looking up towards the Star of Bethlehem, a throng of elated shepherds around her. As the music later swells into the higher registers, 'Then shall the eyes of the blind be opened . . .' the film depicts several scenes of Christ healing the suffering by laying on hands, followed by enigmatic images of happiness: a blinking eye, a smiling face, a young boy throwing down a crutch. After the crucifixion, as the bass aria of Composition XL begins, 'Why do the nations so furiously rage together?', the audience is greeted by a battle scene replete with soldiers in the Roman armour of Christ's era. Suddenly a modern battle tank fills the screen; smoke pouring from its turret, its crew frantically trying to escape. The image cuts to a scene of a World War II infantry charge, followed by the image of a Roman legion on parade. The images share symmetry of energy, the soldiers motivated by a common fervour, their faith in their cause equal in every way, but the surreal scenes have no dialogue, no continuity and it is left to the viewer to make the connections, letting their imagination write the storyline.

When it came time to distribute the film, perhaps unsurprisingly Jack couldn't find any takers. Indifferent to his persistence, theatre owners weren't interested. They said no one would sit through the entire film. The music was nice, but people didn't come to the theatre to listen to music. Jack quickly realised he had sunk two years of his life, and his life savings, into a film few people would ever see. Embarrassed by the failure, Jack returned to Michigan to regroup. He rarely talked about the movie debacle with his friends. When he did, he was blunt and honest about his failure. As he later wrote, 'Being a neophyte I lacked the experience and know-how to engage the right people at the right time to produce a quality film. The result was less than mediocre and a dismal failure.'

The movie hadn't worked out as planned, but Jack knew he had given it his best effort. If he was to make a movie again he would be better prepared. Until then, work would have to occupy his energy. He worked at a hospital in Owosso, Michigan for a short time before returning again to Los Angeles to take a job at the Beverly Hills Medical Center. He split his time between the

Center and Pacific Hospital in Long Beach before finally working full time at Pacific. During this time Jack self-published a short book called *Slimericks and the Demi Diet*, in which he laid out the guidelines he invented as a student for the leave-half-your-plate diet, interspersed with humorous Limericks on the subject. Again, this project was largely ignored.

The hospital work wasn't enough to motivate him to wake up in the mornings. There, he was just another doctor doing a job he'd been hired to do. His research was what people noticed. Granted, they weren't yet noticing him for the reasons he wanted, but by the time he had abandoned his movie project, new events had come into play that he thought had radically changed the playing field.

Jack had stopped his death row campaign during the 60s because public opinion was more in favour of banning capital punishment. Jack too was in favour of this development. But now that the death penalty was inexorably returning, Jack felt it was time to find a way of doing it better. After his recent failures, he was convinced this would give him the opportunity to finally make his mark. As he wrote in *Prescription: Medicide*:

> The fact that death rows existed throughout the moratorium was a good sign that a prediction made in my 1960 monograph was on target: the unstoppable pendulum of history would bring with its next swing a resumption of executions. There was no doubt in my mind that the total and permanent abolition of capital punishment is a delusion of wishful sentimentality trying vainly to insulate itself from the harsh realities of human nature. And I was determined to 'pull out all stops' when that swing back gathered momentum.

Though his opponents lambasted him in the 60s, Jack had no doubts that deep down they knew he was right. He realised that it didn't matter what he said or how he said it; if time was not of the essence, his work would be rejected. As he wrote, 'Ideas succeed not primarily because they are proclaimed, but because their time has come.'

Executions had stopped after two pivotal Supreme Court decisions in 1968 declared the practice unconstitutional, but in the early 70s the Court amended their position to indicate that capital punishment could be used if states were willing to rewrite their death penalty statutes to include more safeguards, such as sentencing guidelines. A number of states quickly passed new death penalty laws, stirring up passionate debate about the death penalty once again. Jack found himself, like many others, particularly drawn to the dramatic Gary Gilmore case in Utah.

Gilmore, a career criminal convicted of murdering a motel manager in Provo, Utah, could have lingered on death row for years, waiting out appeal after appeal, but frustrated by his years spent in prison he clamoured for a quick execution. He took his complaints to the press, being an eloquent and charismatic interviewee, and soon his case was national news. Having successfully stifled his lawyers' efforts to appeal on his behalf, Gilmore was now scheduled to be the first person executed in the US in nearly ten years. The case attracted international attention, with political heavyweights and religious leaders from around the world jostling to be heard. Utah's law offered the condemned two choices of execution, death by hanging or death by firing squad; Gilmore chose firing squad.

As the debate intensified, Jack saw his opportunity. He hoped

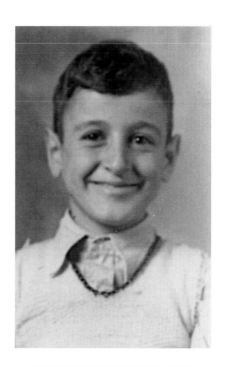

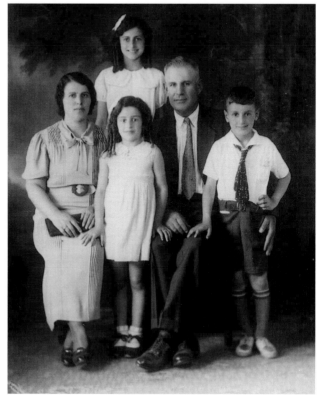

Top:
    Jack, aged seven.

Right:
    Jack, aged eight,
    with his mother,
    Satenig, sisters
    Margo (back)
    and Flora (front),
    and father,
    Levon, 1936.

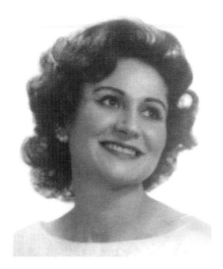

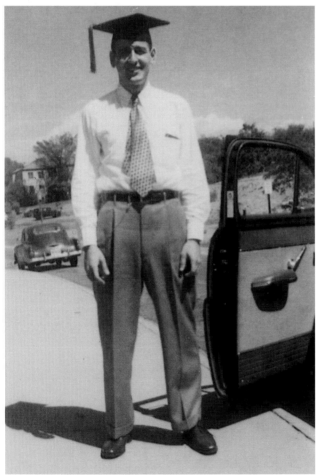

Top:
   Margo, 1944.

Left:
   Jack's high
   school
   graduation
   photo, 1946.

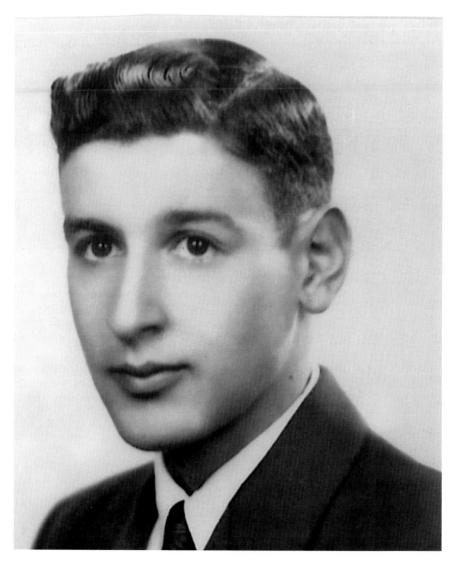

Jack on graduation from medical school, 1952.

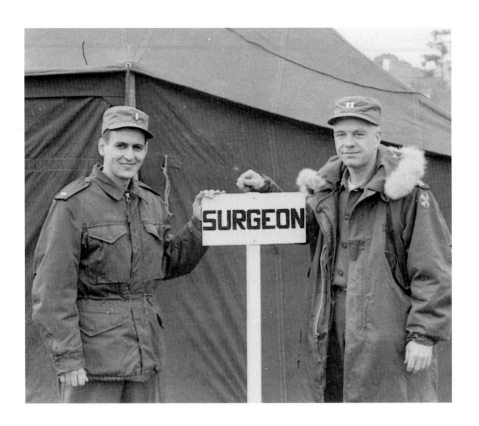

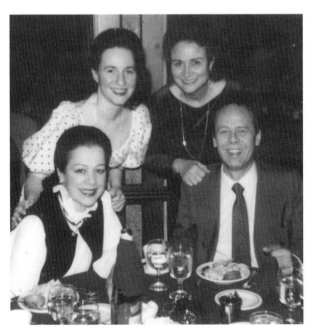

Above:
  Jack as medical
  intelligence officer
  and assistant to
  Dr (Captain)
  LeTellier in Korea,
  1954.

Left:
  Flora, Flora's
  daughter Ava Janus,
  Margo, and Flora's
  husband Herman
  Holzheimer, 1989.

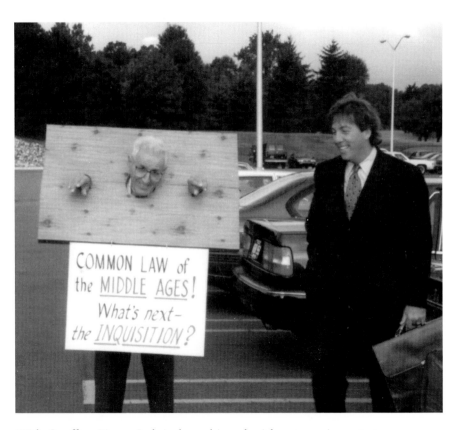

With Geoffrey Fieger. Jack is dressed in colonial costume in protest about being tried by centuries-old common law in May 1996.

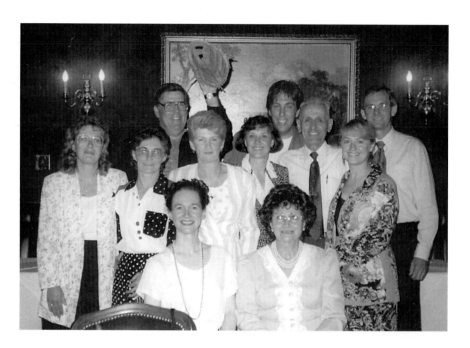

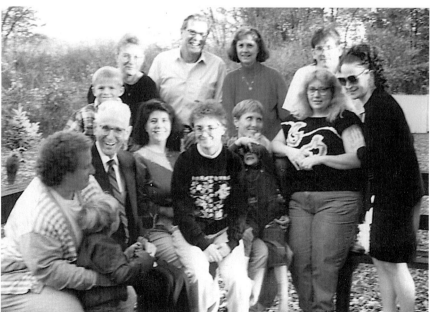

Top:
  'The Survivors', with Neal Nicol and
  Geoffrey Fieger (back row), April 1993.

Bottom:
  'The Survivors' and Jack, June 1994.

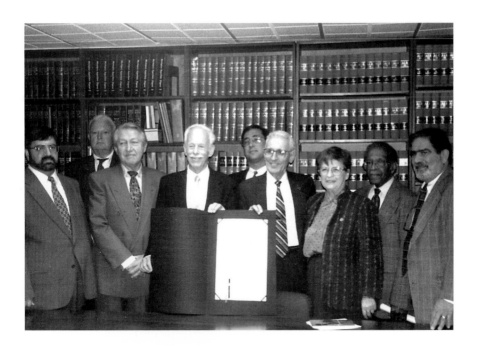

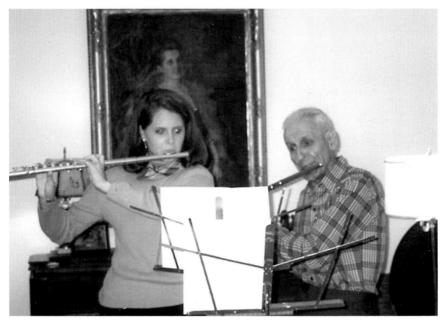

Top:
  With the Physicians of Mercy, October 30th, 1995.

Bottom:
  Jack playing the flute with Sarah Holmes.

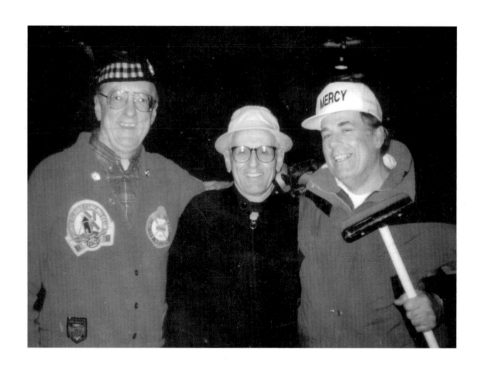

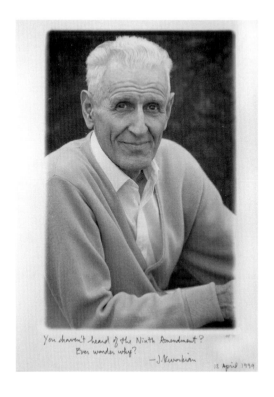

You haven't heard of the Ninth Amendment?
Ever wonder why?
—J. Kevorkian
12 April 1999

Above:
  Harry Wylie, Jack and
  Neal Nicol at the Detroit
  Curling Club, 1998.

Left:
  Jack Kevorkian, 1999.

to persuade Utah authorities to give Gilmore a third option: death through surgical anaesthesia, with the possibility of experimentation or organ transplant. It seemed to Jack like the perfect compromise. Utah would get the vengeance it sought, but Gilmore's life wouldn't be completely wasted. Jack contacted Gilmore's lawyer to see what could be arranged. The lawyer saw the sense in the plan, but after talking about the proposal with Gilmore, he told Jack that Gilmore wasn't interested. He wanted a 'messy' death that would 'scream' in the headlines. Death by anaesthesia simply wouldn't do it in his opinion. Stunned, Jack could only sit back and wait for events to play out.

Gilmore was soon granted his wish, courtesy of a Utah firing squad and four well-aimed bullets. Though Jack felt saddened by the wasted opportunity, he quickly began gathering his old death penalty papers. He hadn't been able to convince Gilmore, but there would be many more convicts to talk to in the years ahead. With vengeance in vogue, people would be ready to hear again Jack's ideas for a better death.

As Jack wrote:

> I learned another hard lesson: erudite articles ceremoniously buried in genteel academic journals did little or nothing (mostly the latter) for the advancement of my campaign. Therefore, I decided that the incubation period had gone on far too long. The time had come to transform my almost ludicrous one-man campaign into more of the mass movement needed to nudge and guide a smugly complacent society … But, how to go about it, and whom to enlist? Corrections and prison officials were resistant; one warden in West Virginia went as far as stating his concern that recipients may

manifest the same traits as the condemned donor. Medical authorities were appalled. Theologians were somewhat aloof and split. And legislators were mute or evasive ... It became apparent that the pressure had to well up from the cellar of society: from a lone doctor at the bottom rung of his calling, without authority, influence, or organisational support (and ultimately even without a job) combined with the absolute lowest of the low, the condemned criminals themselves ... I would have to contact as many death row inmates as possible in order to put together a chorus of voices – the voices that really count – which couldn't help but be heard and perhaps even heeded.

Jack sent numerous letters to convicts in the next few years, taking polls and gathering data that he could make use of in his articles. By 1984 he quit working at the Long Beach hospital primarily because it didn't offer good research possibilities and he required more time for his crusade to change the way America approached capital punishment. He used the seventh floor snack shop of the Long Beach hospital as his 'office', writing a series of articles and letters concerning the death penalty and organ donation, only occasionally pausing for a quick bite of a doughnut while he stared out at the majestic *Queen Mary* anchored across the street.

When he wasn't in his 'office', Jack, now 56 years old, spent his time working from his tiny apartment above a garage on Termino Avenue. His time working as a doctor within the confines of a hospital had effectively ended, and with his retirement he had time to focus on articles and research relating to the end of life. His time in Long Beach would also ultimately mark the end of his anonymity. The work he researched there would lead to his eventual fame.

Though Jack received some support from the prisoners, politicians continued to balk at implementing even the most minor of his suggestions. Some even argued that execution through anaesthesia presented a troubling moral dilemma, and, without further elaborating on how or why, flatly stated that execution by electric chair or hanging was the best option available.

Although it didn't surprise Jack that politicians would continue to stifle his efforts without providing any defence for the flawed system in place, it infuriated him when other doctors began to side against him, stating that it was unethical for any doctor to be involved in any procedure where death was an expected result. Jack fought back the only way he knew how, with his writing.

In subsequent articles, he tried to make his point as clearly as possible. In his eyes, capital punishment was relentless. Though its use had fluctuated through the ages, there had never been a recorded time when capital punishment had completely stopped; that alone was evidence that the desire for capital punishment sprung from the core of the human psyche, and thus could never be eradicated. Jack felt since capital punishment would forever be a part of human history, it was imperative that scientists and philosophers honestly evaluate the benefits mankind wanted to reap from executions, and find the best way to achieve them. Society thought that executions served two primary purposes: to deter future crimes and to punish the criminal. Deterrence was a flawed argument as there was never any clear evidence that capital punishment had any effect as a deterrent to crime. The argument that execution was an effective punishment seemed ever more flawed. As Jack wrote:

> Punishment means the infliction of pain or distress, either physical or mental; but the corpse can experience nothing ... the only possibility of punishment with regard to the death penalty can be the distress caused by the anticipation of being killed and the anxiety over the method selected to do the killing, both of which the penalty (the supposed punishment) immediately relieves! We have here the nonsensical paradox of supreme punishment that punishes only if it is not inflicted.

The truth was that current incarnations of capital punishment didn't have the effect society wanted. Executions would only affect the criminal being executed, thereby solely deterring that particular criminal from committing another crime.

Jack wrote that the true aim of capital punishment was retribution, but that society had turned this into a euphemism for revenge. If retribution was what was desired, then, by definition, capital punishment needed to be honed so that it delivered real compensation or something of value. The involuntary death of a criminal didn't fit that definition – there was no compensation to society other than the loss of a criminal life.

Jack wrote:

> Insincere philosophising obscures the real motive underlying most, if not all, judicial killing: plain revenge, and frequently the more brutal and agonising the better ... The puny advance that lethal injection might be said to represent from a physical standpoint cannot begin to balance the abysmal void it nev-

ertheless sustains ... the backsliding of modern society in this regard is obvious. We wantonly squander priceless opportunities to study ourselves and our living brains, as well as new ways to make us wiser, healthier, and happier. Worse yet, in our 'most enlightened' way of serving justice, we don't even think about making the attempt. So we sanctimoniously keep snuffing out the lives of criminals, many of whom acknowledge their transgression and sincerely desire to somehow make amends. They are eager to give society real retribution by donating their organs and by helping science unlock some of nature's deepest secrets by submitting to otherwise impossible experimentation. But society will not allow it, and doctors refuse to accept it. In callously overriding the personal autonomy of the condemned by denying them the privilege of choice, we inflict on them the worst kind of suffering – far more agonising than any physical pain – the crushing pain of a tortured mind and turbulent soul denied any hope of requital.

Jack's passionate arguments, however, only seemed to find an audience with criminals on death row and the occasional overseas medical journal. The noted Israeli editor Judge Amnon Carmi published Jack's work in a respected international journal *Medicine and Law*, where it was positively received. Within the US, the medical community continued to ignore Jack. Editors of prestigious American medical journals rejected his articles as being too controversial, even though they claimed to be open forums for discussion of such issues. Jack felt he was victim of a concerted effort to silence him. When he was rejected by the *New England Journal of Medicine,* the most prestigious journal of them all, it seemed to him that the rejection was a clear contravention of the journal's own policy to 'offer thoughtful commentary on social, economic, legal, and ethical issues facing the profession', and to be 'an open forum responsive to responsible opinion on all sides of an issue'. The journal brushed him off as an eccentric.

Jack next tried to send a summary of his death penalty proposal to the *Journal* as a letter to the editor, but was rejected because the journal claimed it had a limited amount of space for correspondence and needed 'to present a representative selection of the material received'. The rejection only solidified Jack's feeling that he was being blacklisted.

Repeatedly, the only argument the medical community used in dismissing his proposals was that they violated the Hippocratic oath. Jack found their objections laughable. The medical community already conveniently ignored the Hippocratic oath whenever it suited them, violating at least seven of the roughly ten points of the oath on a regular basis. The oath bans doctors from using the knife, yet doctors routinely perform surgery. Doctors were also supposed to revere their teachers as their parents, and to share their money with them, and keep all elements of medical knowledge secret from anyone except another who had taken the Hippocratic oath.

The most recent example of the medical community adjusting its principles was when the Supreme Court legalised abortion. Jack found it ironic that though the Hippocratic oath explicitly stated 'I will not give to a woman an abortive remedy', doctors now had no problem violating the oath. As he wrote:

> It is clear that the profession has taken the philosophically prudent course of letting public opinion and legal statues

determine whether it is ethical for doctors to perform abortions. Before the 1973 US Supreme Court decision, abortion was illegal and therefore unethical. That decision suddenly made it legal and, of course, ethical; and doctors began doing abortions on a grand scale. Now, will a reversal of the Court's decision make abortion unethical again? Can genuine ethics be so chimerical, so fickle, so aimlessly – almost recklessly – changeable, like the mentality of some scatter-brained child?

The medical community, it seemed to Jack, had no problem redefining ethical behaviour, so long as it could keep doctors like Jack from upsetting their routines.

In the US, doctors were still obsessed with defeating death, again, finding flimsy evidence in the Hippocratic oath for their convictions. Though many doctors believed that the Hippocratic oath forbade them from 'doing harm', the truth was that the edict they so proudly threw in Jack's face was actually from a small treatise Hippocrates had written on epidemics, and commanded a doctor 'to do good or to do no harm'. If one actually studied Hippocrates' writing, it became clear that the only enemy of a doctor was disease. They had to do everything in their power to fight disease, but Hippocrates also made it quite clear that this did not mean that a doctor had to valiantly stave off death at all costs. As Jack wrote, 'In quixotically trying to conquer death, doctors all too frequently do no good for their patients' "ease"; but, at the same time, they do harm instead by prolonging and even magnifying patients' disease.'

Jack's crusade to change the way the nation dealt with capital punishment, and the persistent attempt by the medical establishment to silence him, forced him to widen his research in an effort to find more compelling arguments that might persuade his detractors. In 1986 he discovered that euthanasia was being practised in the Netherlands, and he immediately realised that observing how doctors conducted euthanasia would help him fine-tune his own proposals so that they were more palatable to the medical community in the US. Though illegal in the Netherlands at the time, euthanasia was tolerated. Doctors were openly euthanising as many as 10,000 patients a year, ending the agony of patients who were otherwise doomed to a long and painful death. Jack expanded his death row proposal to include experimentation on willing patients opting for euthanasia, and packed his bags for a trip to Amsterdam in the summer of 1987.

When he arrived, Jack was surprised to find that the doctors there were scandalised by his proposal. Since euthanasia was still illegal in the Netherlands, something Jack hadn't realised, the doctors who performed it didn't want to push the procedure into radical territory that might cause them to lose public support. The doctors were perfectly willing to share their experiences with Jack, but when Jack asked the famous anaesthesiologist Dr Pieter Admiraal what would happen if he took his proposal to Dutch authorities, the doctor said, 'They'd hang you!'

Jack's initial disappointment slowly faded the more he talked with the doctors in the Netherlands. Although the country wasn't the research paradise he had imagined, it gave him hope. He realised he was witnessing a much more significant cause, and one that had a chance of being accepted in the States. The medical establishment and the people of the Netherlands had once been as narrow minded as the groups Jack faced in America. They had changed, however, and that meant that the system in America could also change. All it needed was a catalyst. Jack was ready to begin the process. He would not let terminally ill patients – patients like his mother, who had suffered needlessly for so many months – die in pain when he had such a clear solution to offer. He was ready to fight the war that would immortalise him.

Chapter 8

THE BEGINNING OF THE END

Jack returned to Michigan in 1988, and the following year read in a local Detroit paper about David Rivlin, a 38-year-old quadriplegic in a nursing home in South East Michigan. Rivlin had suffered a spinal-cord injury. He could not move either his arms or his legs nor could he breathe on his own without the assistance of a respirator. Rivlin yearned for independent living. The state of Michigan, however, granted him only $300 a month for support – nowhere near enough to hire the aides he needed – so he ended up in a nursing home (which, ironically, cost the state $230 a day). After three years, Rivlin said he had had enough, and asked to be disconnected from his respirator. The nursing home doctor refused to do so. Rivlin was to eventually get a court order authorising the doctor to sedate him and take him off the ventilator.

Kevorkian went to visit Rivlin in the nursing home before the court order and later described how he had to be turned and fed and have 'everything done for him'. He saw Rivlin as a highly intelligent man who had decided that his life now had no meaning. Jack thought that taking him off his respirator was a cruel way for him to die; he determined to find a better way to help people like Rivlin carry out their own wishes. What he came up with was a suicide machine.

Kevorkian went to a Salvation Army resale store, one of his favourite places to shop, and purchased $3 worth of odds and ends, including a discarded Erector Set with an electric motor and a child's jewellery chain. Within a week he had constructed his Rube Goldberg suicide device. He initially dubbed it the thanatron, which means 'death machine' in Greek, but soon changed its name to the mercitron. A frame for the motor was constructed from Erector beams and the motor mandrel was extended to allow the chain to wind around it like an anchor winch on a boat.

There were three fluid bottles, one for a saline solution, one for Seconal and a third for potassium chloride. Each bottle was directly connected to a single IV line in the patient's arm. The saline solution was to be used as a carrier and to keep the vein open. The Seconal was to sedate the patient and the potassium chloride was used to interrupt the body's electrical signals and stop the heart. There were two steps to the process:

1. Dr Kevorkian would begin the saline IV drip.
2. The patient would flip a switch, which would do two things: First, it would start a solution of Seconal flowing, which would sedate the patient within 20 seconds, and second, it would start a winding process with the chain that acted as a timer. When the chain was fully wrapped around the mandrel, it would trigger the start of the flow of potassium chloride. The patient was fully unconscious at this stage.

With the thanatron/mercitron, death would be fast, absolutely painless – and self-induced.

In the summer of 1989, before Jack got a chance to use his machine, Rivlin was moved from the nursing home to a private home in Ann Arbor. Although the exact details of his death are unknown, it is presumed that his doctors followed the court order and disconnected Rivlin's life support. Food and water was withheld until he died – a practice that is not considered inhumane or illegal by the US judicial system.

Jack still believed that his suicide machine was a viable solution for other people in Rivlin's situation, if only they knew about it. In September 1989, the Oakland County Medical Society turned down Jack's request to advertise the mercitron in its journal. He also wanted to place display ads in several local newspapers, but they turned him down as well (one paper did accept an ad that Jack placed for 'death counselling'). They did find the idea newsworthy, however, and reports of Dr Kevorkian and his suicide machine began to appear in Michigan newspapers and in news services across the country.

In the meantime, Jack began to think about the ramifications of using his machine. He needed to draw up parameters for its use – or for any assisted suicide that anyone else might perform. He did not want anyone to profit by performing this service. Therefore he drew up a series of questionnaires and imperatives for both physicians and patients to follow.

1. Foremost, the patient had to express a firm, voluntary and unwavering wish to die.
2. Medical doctor participation was, and is, a necessity.
3. Implicit medical history was attained.

4. Consultation with family doctors and doctor specialists was a high priority.

5. Extensive and multiple consultations were made, including nearest relatives and/or best friends in attendance, when appropriate and feasible.

6. Psychiatric consultation was required to determine mental competency and lack of any psychiatric disorder.

7. Consultation regarding social interplay was necessary to detect personal or family disputes or irregularities, enabling a clarification of any financial problems among family members.

8. If requested by the patient, clergy was involved.

9. The service was pro bono, free, thereby eliminating any abuse for pecuniary gains.

10. Legal consultation regarding testimonials was recommended.

In other words, the patient must be adamant, incurable, suffering and terminal. Jack felt that only a physician should be allowed to conduct this service, and it should be done free of charge. The physician must always study the patient's medical history and verify the diagnosis and prognosis. The physician should also confer with the patient's family and lawyers to be sure there were no monetary or legal conflicts of interest. Patients should be urged to consult their clergy; if a patient was religious but had no specific minister in mind, the physician should make sure that the patient met with a theologian of the denomination or sect of their choice. The physician must determine (with psychiatric consultation) that the patient is mentally competent to make the decision to end his or her life.

A model of his imperatives was published in the *American Journal of Forensic Psychiatry*, Volume 13, Issue 1, 1992. In the same issue, Jack conveyed his ethical and moral values. He felt that physicians, committed to preserving life at all costs, sometimes overrode patients' autonomy and not only caused pain and suffering, but also magnified it to horrendous proportions. He also felt that this commitment was encouraged by laws that threatened harsh punishment for any physician who, in suitable cases, would want to help end a 'hopelessly tortured life'. He did not believe that every doctor should choose to or be allowed to perform euthanasia or medicide – he thought it should be a specialty, like psychiatry or microsurgery. He envisioned suicide clinics staffed by salaried employees, as opposed to fee-for-service, so that there would be no profit motive. Medicine, Jack felt, was a purely secular profession, and should not be influenced by religion. To him, it was as absurd for a theologian to dictate medical ethics as it was for a doctor to dictate religious ethics.

In addition to his imperatives, Jack developed twelve separate forms he called the 'Fail-Safe Model for Justifiable Medically-Assisted Suicide', designed to regulate the activity and well-being of patient, doctor, hospital and societal security. His twelve forms included:

1. Request for Medically-Assisted Suicide/Final consent for assistance (Witnessed by two doctors)
2. Patient Data (To include family members)
3. Initial Clinical Assessment (Hospital Records and Doctor (Obitiatrist) Examination)
4. Joint Consultation (Interview with patient and all family members)

5. 1st Consultant Report/Review of Patient (Psychiatrist)

6. 2nd Consultant Report/Review of Patient (Sociologist)

7. 3rd Consultant Report/Review of Patient (Neurologist)

8. 4th Consultant Report/Review of Patient (Clergy)

9. 5th Consultant Report/Review of Patient (Psychiatrist, second and confirming)

10. Final Joint Consultation (Patient; Family Only; Patient & Family)

11. Advisory (Five consulting physicians)

12. Final Action (Euthanasia administered)

An example (overleaf) of one form Jack used was published in the *American Journal of Forensic Psychiatry*.

Jack purposely used names like patient Wanda Endittal not only to illustrate the roles involved but to normalise the procedure, and a little light humour seemed a good way to achieve this goal. It didn't have the required effect on his detractors. They thought it was more macabre than funny.

Back in 1989, after several articles had appeared about the Kevorkian suicide machine, *Newsweek* picked up the story. That story was in turn read by three prospective 'patients'. Jack received one letter from the family of a man who was in a coma; Jack turned them down because the man did not have the ability to utilise the mercitron by himself. He was then contacted by a woman he ultimately determined was mentally ill and therefore not able to make an end-of-life decision. His third plea came from Janet and Ron Adkins.

Janet Adkins lived with her stockbroker husband in an affluent Portland, Oregon suburb. Then 54, she had always been active

AMERICAN JOURNAL OF FORENSIC PSYCHIATRY, VOLUME 13, NUMBER 1, 1992 / 33

FIGURE 6

E · MICHIGAN OBITIATRY–ZONE 1 · E

No. 92-1

Consultant Report

CONFIDENTIAL

Patient's Name ___WANDA ENDITTAL___   Age 45   Sex F

Address 1234 Main St., Sumtown, MI 48000   Phone (313) 200-1992

Request   To: Lotte Goode, MD, Psychiatrist   Obitiatrist   Will B. Reddy, MD

     For: Evaluation of mental state and   (Signature) *Will B. Reddy, MD.*

     capability for rational   Date 21 JAN. 1992   Time 9:00 am

     decisions.

Patient   *Wanda Endittal*   Date *1/16/92*   Start Time *1:00 pm*

Site of Consultation *Neuropsychiatric Clinic, City Gen. Hospital, Sumtown, MI*

Consultant's Report:

    Appropriately dressed, middle-aged, severely crippled woman, appears to be mentally alert. Fully oriented as to time, place, person. No concentration deficit. Reasoning and judgment intact (10 out of 10 on Goldfarb Mental Status Exam). No evidence of aphasia. No deficit on Revised Wechsler Memory Scale.

    No evidence of morbid depression, but patient's keen insight into the implications of her progressive neurologic deterioration and incapacity leaves her vulnerable to more severe adjustment reaction with deepening depression.

Conclusion: *Patient is mentally competent and able to come to a rational decision. Mild reactive depression.*

Consultant (Print) *Lotte Goode, MD*   (Signature) *Lotte Goode, MD.*

                                           End Time *3:00 pm*

Review by Patient

Patient's Comments: (DICTATED)

    "I DON'T FEEL DEPRESSED AT ALL."

Site 1234 MAIN ST., SUMTOWN, MI   Date 6 FEB. 1992   Time 5:10 pm

Witness' Signature *Frank Lee Endittal*   Patient's Signature *Wanda Endittal* and energetic – she had raised three successful sons, had been a school teacher, had climbed Mount Hood, Oregon and had gone hang gliding. She also had Alzheimer's disease, a devastating incurable illness that slowly robs individuals of their brain function and imposes an enormous financial and emotional burden upon family and caregivers. For several months, Jack discussed the case with Janet's doctor in Portland, who was against Janet's decision to end her life. He told Jack that she had many years of life ahead of her. Janet's concern, however, was that the longer she waited, the less likely it would be that she would be able to communicate her desires. Jack recommended that Janet enroll in an Alzheimer's research programme. She did, but eventually discovered that the programme had not helped her. That is when she made the decision to go to Michigan with her husband Ron and a friend of theirs to meet with Jack. He conducted four interview sessions (three of which were tape recorded), in which Janet's medical history was discussed, medical records were provided and seven pages of Jack's detailed questionnaire were completed.

At dinner one evening, Jack carefully explained the procedure to Janet, Ron and their friend. Although she was becoming forgetful, Janet could still carry on a conversation and was well aware of the fate that awaited her as a victim of Alzheimer's. She willingly signed the papers Jack gave her.

For two days Jack scouted locations to perform the medicide. He didn't want to use his own apartment out of fear that if his landlord found out he might be evicted. He was turned down by several motels, funeral homes and the landlords of vacant office space. Eventually, he decided that the only available place was the inside of his Volkswagen van. He bought curtains for the windows and installed a cot which he made up with new sheets and pillowcases. On a beautiful day in June, Ron and Janet's friend said their goodbyes at the hotel at which the three had been staying and remained behind while Jack, Janet and Jack's sister Flora drove to the nearby Groveland Oaks campgrounds. In the van, Dr Kevorkian hooked Janet up to an electrocardiograph machine so he could monitor her heart, and then attached her to the mercitron. Her last word to Jack was, 'Hurry.' Respecting her Christian faith, Jack's response was, 'Safe journey.'

Less than six minutes later, the line on the heart monitor was flat. Jack disconnected Janet from the machines, then called the police and told them what he had done.

The police arrived on the scene and immediately arrested, arraigned and incarcerated Jack. They confiscated his van and the mercitron. However, Michigan didn't have a law against assisted suicide – so technically Jack had committed no crime. No charges were filed, and he was released from custody.

The following evening, Ron Adkins and two of his three sons held a press conference back in Portland, where they read from a suicide note Janet had written hours before her death. The note said:

> I have decided for the following reasons to take my own life. This is a decision taken in a normal state of mind and is fully considered. I have Alzheimer's disease and I do not want to let it progress any further. I do not want to put my family or myself through the agony of this terrible disease.

In an interview the *New York Times* on June 6th, 1990, Kevorkian stated: 'My ultimate aim is to make euthanasia a positive experience. I'm trying to knock the medical profession into accepting its responsibilities, and those responsibilities include assisting patients with death.' He also said that he took the action partly to 'force the medical and legal establishment to consider his ideas.'

The *Times* also interviewed Judith R Ross, a professor of medical ethics at the University of California at Los Angeles, who stated there was a thin line between withdrawing care (as was done in the Rivlin case) and actually giving a patient something that will cause his or her death. She acknowledged, however, that the thin line was 'being nudged every day' as doctors often surreptitiously gave patients the means to kill themselves. 'It's not uncommon,' she said, 'for physicians of cancer patients to say, "Here's some medication and make sure you don't take more than 22 pills because 22 pills will kill you."'

Shortly after Janet Adkins' death, the Alzheimer's Association issued a statement (which can now be found on their website):

> We are very saddened by the tragic case of Janet Adkins. We believe that hers was a very personal decision; however, we must also affirm the right to dignity and life for every Alzheimer patient and cannot condone suicide.
>
> This tragedy epitomised the desperation that individuals with Alzheimer's disease and their families feel when the diagnosis is Alzheimer's — an incurable disease. We hope that the discussion surrounding the Janet Adkins case will help stimulate further action on the part of the federal government to support research into discovering the cause of this devastating illness and, therefore, prevent such desperate acts.
>
> It is tragic that Janet Adkins chose to take her life. We want others in her situation to know that there are services and

programs to assist such patients and families in coping with Alzheimer's disease, and we encourage them to seek professional help.

The association also asserted that assisted suicide and euthanasia are not the same as refusing or withdrawing treatments and that:

> When treatment is withheld or withdrawn, the intent is not to kill but to unburden the person from a technological assault on a natural dying. If the person lives on, he or she will still be cared for well and attentively, often with a hospice philosophy, which focuses on providing comfort and treating pain.
>
> The Association asserts that the refusal or withdrawal of any and all medical treatment is a moral and legal right for all competent Americans of age. This right can be asserted by the competent patient in legal documents concerning end-of-life care or by a family surrogate acting on the basis of either 'substituted judgment' (what would the patient have wanted) or 'best interests' (what seems the most humane and least burdensome option in the present).

Jack considered these tenets to be both hypocritical and inhumane. He felt the refusal or withdrawal of treatment could be construed to be the same as a death sentence, only with the addition of cruel and unusual punishment. The stricken will surely die, but in a prolonged, possibly anguished process for the patient, the caregivers and loved ones. Additionally, he questioned from what fount would the palliative care be drawn? Medicare and Medicaid were overburdened. Insurance companies did not acknowledge the terminal diagnosis of Alzheimer's. Hospice care was provided for the last six months of a patient's life but no one could determine the lifespan of an Alzheimer's patient. Who is to pay for the 24-hour care required for the patient up to this mystic six-month prognostication? Where will the money come from? Where will the love, understanding and continued patience come from?

In 1998, when the assisted-suicide controversy was in the headlines again due to Jack's trial for the death of Thomas Youk, the Alzheimer's Association published a letter from Ron Adkins explaining the decision his wife had made:

> My wife, Janet Adkins was excited by life. She was a woman of many ideas and interests. She was a talented musician and an avid reader. She liked pushing the limit and trying new things, such as trekking to Nepal.
>
> When she was diagnosed with Alzheimer's disease at age 53, she was devastated. She weighed the opinions of letting the disease take her mind and body or exiting early with the assistance of a doctor while her intellect was still intact. We had openly discussed end-of-life issues, and her choice was not to let the disease progress.
>
> We made an informed decision and a personal choice, one that was right for Janet. Most importantly we opened end-of-life issues together as a family. I encourage others to do the same.

It seemed some lessons had been learned. The Alzheimer's Association then asserted:

While the furor surrounding physician-assisted suicide has the potential to polarize American society, the debate has also focused the Alzheimer's Association on improving end-of-life services ... More importantly, the creation of such options will help reduce the suffering and grief associated with the final stages of Alzheimer's disease.

Because of Jack, many people with this dreaded disease are living – and dying – with more grace and dignity.

Chapter 9

THE HELPERS AND THE HELPED

The picture of Jack Kevorkian most people have in their minds is of an obsessed loner who single-handedly set out to change the laws of the land on assisted suicide. In some ways that picture is correct. Like Don Quixote, Jack often tilted at windmills and fought his battles with a determination and purpose others could not even comprehend.

But Jack did not go into battle alone. Even Don Quixote had his faithful companion Sancho Panza, and Jack had several faithful, loyal and courageous companions of his own.

Jack's two biggest supporters were his sisters. When their mother was dying they were at her bedside every day, pleading with the doctors to help end her suffering. They had seen the devastation first hand, and it fuelled their efforts to help Jack in his cause.

Flora assisted Jack with all the details of Janet Adkins' medicide. When she returned to Germany soon after to be with her husband, Margo – the matriarch of the family since their mother's death – took over. It was a task she relished and took on with fervour and tenacity. She was a retired executive assistant from Chrysler who quickly rose through the ranks because of her attention to detail, her typing expertise, her tireless energy and her winning smile. These attributes stood her in good stead for creating and collating the myriad of forms that Jack's obitiatry practice generated. Married and divorced, with one daughter, she acted as chauffeur, confidante, patient advocate, sounding board, counsellor and videographer, which earned her the nickname of Cecil, for the great pioneer of the film industry Cecil B DeMille. She was frequently the main contact with the patients and their families, doing all the letter writing and reviewing of requests, and often held the patient's hand during the procedure. She was a special solace for female patients. She comforted the families while the patient was undergoing the procedure and often even after the event. She was Jack's only conspicuous female companion, his invaluable ally and his strongest supporter.

It was Margo who brought Geoffrey Fieger into the fold. Although Jack had not faced any charges for the Adkins medicide, he was initially arraigned before District Court Judge Gerald McNally, who advised him to obtain legal counsel. Margo had read about a brash young lawyer who was, at the time, collecting an award owed him by a local hospital. When payment was not forthcoming, Fieger began to collect furniture and computers from their offices. Fieger was promptly paid what he was due. Margo was impressed; she contacted Fieger and she and Jack went to see him.

Geoffrey was (and is) as flamboyant as one could imagine. He is six foot five, raw boned, ruggedly handsome, with unruly collar-length rusty hair. He is an 'in your face' lawyer whom the police and many other lawyers dread to encounter. At the time Geoffrey met

Margo and Jack, he was a relatively unknown lawyer who adulated his well-known labour activist parents, his rock star brother Doug and his accomplished author sister Beth.

Fieger majored in drama at the University of Michigan prior to law school – a bent which has certainly held him in good stead throughout his career. He has had his own radio show and television series, and is now a frequent guest and legal expert for several media outlets. He is an immensely talented trial attorney. However, it was his pro bono services for Jack Kevorkian and his cause that made him a nationally known and highly sought after legal eagle.

Fieger was also a big fan of Jack's sister Margo. He has said:

> Margo had more to do with Jack's adventures, and control thereof, than any other human being. No one had a more powerful influence on Jack Kevorkian than Margo, nobody, except perhaps his parents. She was Jack's older sister and the only person he would really trust; a surrogate parent in a way. She was his common sense because Jack doesn't have any common sense. Jack is a brilliant, brilliant, guy but has very little, if any, common sense. If given the choice in terms of doing tactical things, which is amazing because he thinks he's a tactician, he will always go awry. In terms of his understanding of at least what was going on around him during the maelstrom of the assisted suicide debate, he had little understanding of it, or little understanding of his importance in the big picture, which as events unfolded was probably a good thing. Jack was really on a freefall and he probably wouldn't be in prison today if Margo were alive. When she passed, Jack was rudderless, and henceforth unheeded my counsel.

One can't understand Jack without understanding the influence of his family, of Margo. He would have gone down, self-destructed at the very beginning of his assisted suicide journey, as he later did, had it not been for Margo's positive, insightful and stabilising influence. He would not have retained me as his lawyer, he wouldn't have gone along with the things I did to promote and create a national debate.

In what must have been a devastating example of Jack's working against his own best interest, he and Margo had a bitter disagreement one night in the summer of 1992. They were having dinner in a local Big Boy restaurant on their way to videotape a consultation with a patient, and Margo made a comment to which Jack took offence (a comment which no one present now remembers). Margo held her ground, and Jack escalated the argument. It got very loud. Margo got up from the table, went out to her car, brought in the camera and handed it to Jack, and then left for home. She never helped Jack again, and she died of a heart attack six months later at the age of 68.

'Margo, although she was very supportive and sometimes may have even encouraged him where he didn't want to go, nonetheless had a civility about her, a kindness about her,' said the Rev Ken Phifer, a Unitarian minister in Ann Arbor who helped a member of his own church arrange a Kevorkian-assisted suicide. 'Jack lost his better half when he lost Margo.'

One of the witnesses to the incident at the Big Boy was Jack's old friend Neal Nicol, who had come back into the picture in 1991. Neal hadn't seen Jack for about 15 years, but having heard about Jack's exploits through the media he left his business card at his apartment in Royal Oak offering to assist him in any manner possible. Kevorkian immediately called – not to say hello and reminisce about old times, but to ask if he could use Neal's home for further medicides. He was getting too much flack about campgrounds and his rusty old VW van. Neal was separated from his wife and renting an apartment and like Jack couldn't take the chance of getting evicted. Neal suggested hospitals, funeral homes and churches, but they would not take the risks involved.

By this time Michigan state regulators had suspended Jack's medical licence and he could not legally attain Seconal, so Jack had evolved a second method of assisting his patients using carbon monoxide. First, a mask was placed over the patient's nose and mouth, connected via a tube to a cylinder of the deadly gas. Next, a valve was released to start the gas flowing. If it was too difficult for a patient to turn the valve, a clip or a clothespin was clamped onto the tubing and pulled off to allow the gas to flow. Because this process sometimes took as long as ten minutes, Jack often suggested that patients take sedatives to keep them calm throughout.

When the police learned about Jack's carbon monoxide purchase, they threatened the supplier who succumbed to pressure and refused further sales. Jack then researched the chemical manufacture of CO and asked Neal, who then had his own laboratory supply company, if he could get the ingredients: calcium carbonate and zinc powder. Neal said he could, and did just that. He soon realised that just because Jack could no longer get CO canisters, it didn't mean that he couldn't – so he began purchasing supplies for Jack. Neal proved so useful that at one point Jack naïvely asked if he knew any drug dealers. He thought Neal could simply go downtown and buy all the barbiturates and downers they needed from nefarious drug dealers.

Once Neal's divorce became final he bought a home in Waterford, Michigan. Jack now had a serene, clinical site for his burgeoning avocation. Neal wanted to make sure his neighbours would not be upset once they found out what he was doing. He canvassed the neighbourhood and found that they were sympathetic and supportive. After Margo died, Neal took over the videotaping of the consultations, the clerical work and the patient contacts.

Neal's first, and Jack's fifth, patient was a terminally ill woman of 52, Lois Hawes. She had the blessing of her family and, most significantly, the support of her physicians. The physicians consulted included Lois's family practitioner, her cancer specialist, an internist and a number of radiologists. They also provided Jack with her medical records. She was suffering excruciating pain from lung cancer that had spread to her brain and she was given only three months to 'live'. Her four sons and a niece attended the passing.

Neal said he was surprised at his own clinical reaction to the procedure. It was a non-event for him, but a huge event for Ms. Hawes. He related, 'Not to appear crass, but the decision, the procedure was faultless. She opened the gas line and in two minutes she was peacefully asleep and in five she was gone. She went so peacefully.' If Neal had had any doubts about his participation before this, they were now gone for good.

In 1994 Jack found another able helper in Janet Good, who was then president and founder of the Michigan chapter of the Hemlock Society (which became End of Life Choices and eventually merged with another group to become Compassion and Choices). The Hemlock Society, founded by Derek Humphrey in 1980, was the first organised right-to-die society in the United States.

Janet became involved with the society because she spent three years caring for her own ailing mother in the mid-1970s, watching a healthy, feisty woman languish in agony. Janet was a wonderful, caring, defiant lady whose eleventh commandment was 'Thou shall not standby and do nothing.'

The Hemlock Society presidency and counsellor to Jack Kevorkian were not Janet's first or only pioneering endeavours. In 1991 she was inducted into the Michigan Women's Hall of Fame. The acknowledgement advises:

In 1965, Janet worked against the war on poverty with the Archdiocese of Detroit and then went onto become acting director of Equal Employment Opportunity for the Michigan Employment Security Commission. Co-chairing the Governor's task force on sexual harassment led to the initiative to make sexual harassment an issue in unemployment insurance. The task force was successful in bringing about the inclusion of sexual harassment as an unlawful practice in the Elliott-Larsen Civil Rights Act. Good was the driving force in establishing the Older Women's League (OWL) in Michigan, later becoming its first state president. She also founded and served as president of the Michigan Hemlock Society, the nation's chief right-to-die advocacy organisation. She is active in the Catholic Church as well, serving on the board of Catholics for Choice. Publicly she invited feminists to tithe to feminist causes. Having declared, 'There is nothing more important than women,' Good actively pursues a policy of forming critical social institutions, awareness, and legislation affecting the lives of women.

Fortunately for Jack, Janet was able to replace Margo as his administrative assistant. She left her post with the Hemlock Society and embarked upon this new endeavour with compassion, industry and aptitude. She concerned herself with the logistics of keeping the assisted suicide munificence going. Janet made introductory contacts, prerequisite patient interviews, follow-ups on patient obligations and requirements, attended weekly meetings for candidate selection and ran hither and yon as cases required. She supported Jack in court and at news conferences, speaking to reporters, but for the most part stayed out of the limelight.

While Janet was doing her best to help the ill and injured she developed pancreatic cancer, and was not expected to live beyond three months. She lived for two more years.

Ray Good, Janet's husband, was a Detroit Inspector and Precinct Commander on the force for 28 years and was still on the force when Janet started working with Kevorkian. The Goods had numerous discussions and arguments, like all married couples, but never about what Jack and Janet were doing. Ray really believed in their work. 'We used to get calls day and night with requests for Jack's help,' Ray once said. 'Some people wanted to believe that he was offing people left and right, at will, but I would guess that for every hundred calls we received Jack would maybe, maybe, help one.'

Ray had genuine affection for Jack. They would argue in jest and Ray was proud to be able to hold his own in these verbal combats. Ray has said:

> I think if Janet were alive she would have prevented him from
> doing some of the crap he did. She was an anchor for him, had

great influence on him and perhaps he wouldn't be where he is today if she were around to counsel him.

When it was finally time for Janet to go, all I can say is thank God for the Doc. She was in such pain and the morphine power was running out. Many, many nights she would wake up yelling and seeing things on the wall, having hallucinations like a drunk. The pain was so terrible! It was pathetic to see this strong woman suffer so. It made me cry. There was some sort of governor on the needle plunger that prevented her from giving herself enough medicine, at that time, to give her complete freedom from the pain. I really don't know how it worked, but near the end it really didn't work at all.

God bless Doc.

On August 26th, 1997 – the 77th anniversary of the enactment of the amendment to the US Constitution giving women the right to vote – Janet became one of Dr Kevorkian's patients.

'She was as close as any woman has ever been to Dr Kevorkian,' said Geoff Fieger. 'She was his right hand, his left hand and his conscience. She was really the impetus and moving force behind Dr Jack Kevorkian.'

In a statement read by Fieger, Kevorkian said:

Janet's courage and strength of character far exceeded in quality and quantity that represented by the collective courts and legislatures of this morally benighted country. Janet exemplified the best in women: She fought for freedom, liberty, justice and compassion. I loved her. We all will miss her.

Of course by this time Jack Kevorkian and his campaign for assisted suicide were famous, or infamous, as the case may be. He had been practising assisted suicide for eight years. Michael Schwartz, a partner in Geoffrey Fieger's law firm who represented Jack in several of his court appearances, described Jack's patients' situations:

> Jack's patients were about to end their lives, in the midst of a pretty horrible situation. They could not generally conduct a conversation in a calm, dispassionate manner. They know what is about to happen; they really know that this is 'the end'. Many of the patients were young and didn't have an opportunity to experience life, total life. They were denied that because their one opportunity at life was stolen from them by disease. Every interview, every event was a major tragedy, and Jack knew that, he had great compassion and empathy with his patients. He repeatedly offered them alternatives, but they were steadfast, they knew what they were doing.

After Janet Adkins' death, Jack feared he might be going to jail, but he had already agreed to help Marjorie Wantz and Sherry Miller. He was afraid that if he was incarcerated he might be able to help one but not the other and he suggested that they die together. They agreed. Both Sherry and Marjorie were very vocal about their desire to have Dr Kevorkian help them die. They did a number of media interviews and radio and television appearances, making their decision quite clearly and publicly known.

Sherry Miller was bedridden with multiple sclerosis (MS), a serious chronic and progressive illness affecting the body's nerves, rendering a person disabled. She was 43 years old, single and lived with her parents. She had lost control of all her bodily functions and her parents had to hand feed her. She believed, like many deists, that she would go to heaven because God had not meant for her to suffer as she did. Jack attempted to consult Sherry's MS 'specialist', but was summarily ejected from his office at Henry Ford Hospital.

Marjorie Wantz, 58, although not terminally ill, suffered from excruciating pain. She had gone to a doctor to have benign vaginal tumours removed, but ten operations later she still found herself unable to sleep. Her husband recalled how she would scream through the night, which kept even her neighbours awake. Doctors tried to help, but every blood test and scan returned the same result: there was nothing physically wrong with her. They determined that her pain was psychosomatic, and the psychiatrists she saw agreed. They also agreed that Marjorie Wantz was depressed and suicidal; she had attempted to take her life several times. Then she discovered Dr Kevorkian.

Once she started talking to Jack, she stopped talking to her psychiatrists. At Kevorkian's insistence, she saw a psychiatrist who found her sane and able to make medical decisions. She pursued Jack for several years until he finally agreed to help her commit suicide.

On October 22nd, 1991, one day before their deaths, Dr Kevorkian videotaped a consultation with the two women. During the taping, Wantz admitted that she had tried killing herself several times:

> I tried to ... I put the hose on the exhaust and through the
> window. I stayed in the car over three hours, I tried it three

times. Nothing happened. And my doctor told me within about 25 minutes that's all it should take. I was in there three hours. I didn't get sleepy, I didn't get sick. I felt a little nausea, nothing.

I took 120 … [inaudible] two different times. And I was told well, 120, that's nothing, you need 4,000 of … [inaudible]. So, I've tried everything short of a gun. I've tried loading a gun, but I don't know how to load one. If I did, I probably would have. As [my husband] said, I probably wouldn't have succeeded … And this way I feel it's going to be done right. It's going to be fast, no mistakes. If you did it yourself, you don't know what you're doing. And I've had it for so long, I don't want any more of it.

The videotaping was conducted at the home of Sherry Miller's parents. They were both present, as were Sherry's sister and two brothers. Dr Kevorkian asked her brother Gary how he felt about Sherry's decision:

Gary: My real feelings are that I hate to see my sister kill herself. On the other hand, I have to respect her judgment that says she can decide the quality of her life.

Kevorkian: Would you feel better if she changed her mind and went on a little longer? Be honest.

Gary: I've heard her say this for a long time. And I've had discussions over the years with her. And I've never seen her say, 'Oh, I have hope, things are going to get better. By the way, I plan to get into some form of therapy, or I'm going to pursue meditation.' I've never heard her say, 'I'm holding out hope.' And I've gradually seen her, and maybe me more

than my parents, have seen – because I see her more peri-
odically and so the changes are more dramatic to me. And it
always has been somewhat of a shock when I come back to
Michigan and see that this is not theoretical, this is actually a
degeneration. I think she has the right to say –

Sherry: I've had enough.

Gary: That I've had enough. I could not put the needle in her
arm. I could not hold a pillow over her head. But, I'm not
going to step in and stop her from doing this.

Marjorie Wantz and Sherry Miller died side by side on two cots
in a rustic log cabin in Bald Mountain state recreation area north
of Detroit. Jack had enough Seconal to attend to one patient,
but altered his method to carbon monoxide for the second. He
would have preferred to use the mercitron because of its potential medical acceptance as a medical 'procedure' – doctors love
procedures. He also worried about public aversion to gas, often
due to its connotation with both world wars. He discovered,
however, that his patients didn't care either way, as the carbon
monoxide procedure was as peaceful and foolproof as with intravenous fluids.

When the double medicide was over, Jack once again dialled
911. The police arrived, along with the fire department, newspaper
reporters and television cameras. The local county sheriff took
Jack into custody and confiscated his van and his equipment. This
time, though, Geoffrey Fieger was on hand, and the sheriff didn't
keep Jack or his van for very long.

Once again, the judiciary was faced with a situation they did
not know how to handle. There was still no law against assisted
suicide in Michigan. But later on Jack would be prosecuted (and

persecuted) for the deaths of Marjorie Wantz and Sherry Miller, as well as Thomas Hyde, Merian Frederick, Dr Ali Khalili, Loretta Peabody and Thomas Youk.

Thomas Hyde was locked inside a body that didn't work. He was only 30 years old, living with his girlfriend and their baby daughter. In August 1992, he had come home scared to death. He told his girlfriend that he couldn't coordinate his hands, they wouldn't do what he wanted, preventing him from even holding a hammer. After visiting several doctors and undergoing countless tests, the heart-rending, most dreaded prognosis was confirmed. He had ALS, Lou Gehrig's disease, the debilitating, always-fatal progressive neuromuscular disorder caused by the death of the motor nerve cells that control voluntary muscle movement. The degradation started immediately. When his girlfriend was in the hospital about to give birth to their daughter, her family thought Tom was drunk because his speech was so slurred. Each day he lost a little more control of his own body and within a year he was unable to walk, his speech was almost incomprehensible and he had great difficulty swallowing. Doctors suggested, and he agreed, to attend an ALS support group. This was a big mistake – he now saw first hand what was in store for him. Hospice personnel visited daily to clean and feed him. He decided not to go on with this painful, mortifying, incapacitating disease.

Tom took a trip to Florida to visit his mother. She had recently lost her husband to cancer and it was Tom's hope that she might have some morphine left over from his palliative care. Unfortunately, she didn't. He asked his 22-year-old brother to help him commit suicide but Sean said he couldn't. Tom returned to Michigan and found that he had lost the ability to even lift his infant daughter. On one occasion a friend came to visit and found Tom leaning against his house with dried faeces from waist down. He was trying to reach the garden hose to clean himself off. The friend retrieved the hose and helped, but time couldn't erase the humiliation they both suffered. Tom wrote to Jack Kevorkian.

Jack, Margo and Neal went to Tom's apartment to film the first consultation. Tom's speech was indistinct but the three were able to understand, 'I want to end it, I want to die.' He then broke down and cried. Everyone present shed tears too. His medical records were voluminous because he had enrolled in a research study that had, unfortunately, not helped. A panel of six doctors concurred on his diagnosis. He was facing death by strangulation from his own saliva because soon he would be unable to clear his airway.

Tom was a hunter and loved the great outdoors and wished to die in the open air. Jack and Neal visited parks in the area but decided not to use the common ground because they might run into the police before or during the event. They decided to perform the carbon monoxide medicide in the VW van in Royal Oak behind Jack's apartment. Neal picked Tom up early on the morning of August 4th, 1993, to drive him to Royal Oak. He requested to take one of his prescribed sedatives to calm him before seeing Jack. They stopped on an exit ramp so he could take his pill and while swallowing he choked and spit up water. He tried to say something that was difficult to discern until, after several attempts, Neal understood 'pardon me', and tears were shed again.

After the medicide, Jack drove Tom, deceased in the back of the van, to the beautiful setting of Belle Isle in the Detroit River and left him there to await the police.

★

Merian Frederick was a very venturesome lady. She and her engineering professor husband loved to dance, canoe, sail, swim, read and hike. She was a socially conscious woman involved in her community and church. She protested the Vietnam War in Washington and was actively involved in the nuclear freeze campaign Common Cause and Amnesty International. At her church, she spearheaded a sanctuary for an El Salvadoran refugee family. On one occasion, she and her husband went camping across Europe where they ended up behind the Iron Curtain, tenting in the suburbs of Moscow.

Merian was a loving woman. She instilled love of family, community, country and life into her five children. Friends congregated at their household because it was always vibrant and full of laughter. Merian cared for her husband when he was laid low with colon cancer, which eventually took him from her. She nursed her mother for five years following a debilitating stroke.

In 1989, at the age of 67 Merian was diagnosed with ALS. In the early stages of the disease her speech thickened, she had trouble swallowing and she was continually drooling. In four short years she deteriorated to the point where she couldn't speak at all, and needed a suction machine to remove her saliva. She required a feeding tube for sustenance and a makeshift head support to sit erect.

During these horrific years she used a computer, adaptive telephone devices, and paper and pen to write and sketch. These devices eventually failed her and she could only rely on gestures and abbreviated pen scratches. She went for counsel with her church minister, and before complete debilitation, on September 15th, 1993, she laboriously typed a note to Dr Jack Kevorkian:

I have, I think, preliminary warnings that my trunk and neck muscles will not much longer support my head, and that my upper arms will not allow me to reach more than a few inches from my body. And my forearm begins to tire when typing ... Since I cannot speak, that will mean the end of meaningful communication for me ... do you think you will be able to help me?

Kevorkian went through his customary prerequisites and logged in his notes:

The degree of physical impairment, which seemed to be quite localised to the head and neck, did not seem to me to justify termination of life at this time ... I suggested that the patient seek consultation with regard to a special brace to reinforce neck muscles and keep the head upright ...

The debilitation, however, continued. Her mind was clear, but it was trapped in a body that sabotaged all attempts at communication. Her muscles degenerated to the point where her speech was gone; she could no longer hold her head up and her hands were losing the ability to use her computerised communication system. She did not want to become an active mind imprisoned in a useless body. She couldn't go on.

Merian's notes, prior to her complete physical breakdown, stated:

I see the rest of my life being spent solving all sorts of problems, how to type, how to reach for things, how to eat without being nauseous or constipated, how to hold up my head without a brace that won't gag me, or cause pressure points or 'bed sores' where the brace sits on my skin. How to be strong enough, or get enough breath to sit up for a while, walk a few steps, stand up for a hug. A life of being mindful always of my throat so I don't let it clog up and gag me.

I have two criteria for meaningful existence, (1) a posture that allows me to write without undue fatigue, (2) finger and forearm strength that allow typing and writing.

Other notes expressed:

And why are we spending all this effort? So I can wake up every morning thinking, another day to dread living thru ... But I see life from here on as a losing battle, too many balls in the air, too much effort spent solving the problem of how to stay alive and no energy or time left to do any real living. To sum up, I want out, the earliest, most humane way possible.

Willingness of loved ones to attend to me is heartwarming, but unless some joie de vivre returns I'd just as soon quit while I still have some control over quitting.

She wrote her daughter in California:

If I choose my own time it has to be a time that I find intolerable, while I still have the strength to initiate the action. If I wait until all of you are ready, I would have to live a long time. With five kids and seven grandkids there is never going to be a time when everyone is ready. If I get the nerve to act again – I want to act quickly.

After Jack revisited Merian, he knew she was ready for his service; mentally, medically and religiously.

On her last night, the entire family met to say their goodbyes. The following morning Merian, her son Rick and her pastor drove across Detroit from Ann Arbor to Royal Oak and Dr Kevorkian's apartment. Her minister later recalled that Kevorkian repeatedly asked Merian whether she wanted to go ahead, emphasising that it was her decision. 'Merian, do you have any doubts about your decision about what you want?' She raised her right hand and signalled 'no' then wrote 'NO' in large letters on her pad.

The other patient present that day, together with his wife, was Dr Ali Khalili. A rehabilitation medicine and qualified pain management specialist, and an associate professor at Northwestern University just north of Chicago, Dr Khalili was also there to end his suffering.

In October 1989, aged 57, Dr Khalili slipped on a piece of carpet and put out his arm to stop the fall. He didn't actually fall, but he nonetheless felt excruciating pain in his arm. X-rays determined he had broken his arm but the question was, why? He scheduled a visit to the Mayo Clinic in Rochester, Minnesota – one of the largest and most respected medical institutions in the United States. There he was diagnosed with multiple myeloma, bone cancer.

Back at Northwestern University, the doctor intensely researched multiple myeloma, discussed his condition with specialists in the field, received input from colleagues and became an expert in the area of bone cancer. He discovered that no matter what course of treatment he chose, the outcome would be the same: a long drawn-out painful journey to death that could also include complete paralysis. His colleagues and friends offered little encouragement. In fact, one friend told him, 'Tomorrow will be worse than today and the last thing you want is to live long with this impaired quality of life.'

Ali underwent a conservative course of chemotherapy, one with the least amount of side effects, but also one that would buy him little extra time on earth. In August 1993 he suffered compression fractures of the spine, underwent radiation therapy with minor improvement, had a morphine pump installed, closed his office, bought an electric bed and went home.

During the interview process with Jack Kevorkian, Dr Khalili said, 'The patient is the *only one* that can judge "quality of life". It's an individual decision and the option of euthanasia should be available to everyone.' He regretted that sometimes in the past he had too often dismissed patients' complaints of pain and disability.

Jack asked the obvious question, 'You're a doctor, why don't you do it yourself? You can obtain the medications; you know what has to be done and how to do it. Why not go quietly in your own bed and help retain the illusion of medical omnipotence?' His reply was candid yet refreshing, 'I want a professional to help me, one that can guarantee nothing will go wrong which could leave me worse off than before the assistance.'

On November 22nd, 1993 in his Royal Oak apartment, Dr Jack Kevorkian helped Merian Fredrick and Dr Ali Khalili find peace of mind and a quiet departure.

Loretta Peabody was a 54-year-old sufferer of multiple sclerosis, who was wheelchair bound. She sent a videotape to Jack, pleading for his help and saying that because of her illness, she was turning into a 'vicious, nasty woman'.

'I appreciate your time and your efforts to help people in my situation,' she said. 'There is nothing I can do for myself, and I can't do this any more. I've fought this as long as I could fight it and if it wasn't for you I don't know what I'd do.'

Jack visited her on August 30th, 1996 in Ionia County, Michigan, and made a heart rending consultation tape in which she is shown crying and saying 'thank God you are here', and repeating that she can't go on any more the way she is:

> Jack: What is it that you want to do now?
> Loretta: I want to leave.
> Jack: Isn't there anything in your life worth going on for despite your incapacitation?
> Loretta [crying]: I can't do it any more. I just can't.

Loretta Peabody died that day. Four days later, her family physician ruled that she had died of natural causes. No autopsy was conducted, and her body was cremated.

Not everyone Jack helped was to die. George Murphy, a former assistant prosecutor in Michigan, was like many of the people that contacted Dr Kevorkian. When George broke his knee due to a fall in the tub, he placed his faith – and his money – in the hands of a fellow lawyer. He gave this friend power of attorney and the associate stole George's life savings.

George was 74, lonely, ambulated by walker and in pain. He couldn't drive his car because of an accident caused by an overdose of medication, and he had no one to transport him to and from a pain clinic. He felt that life wasn't worth living, so he gave Kevorkian a call. After listening to his story, Jack and Neal went to see George at his apartmant. Kevorkian's opinion was that he didn't really want to die – he just needed some companionship and some new interests. He told George that what he should do was to control his pain and get on with his life.

Neal kept in touch with George every couple of weeks as his lab had an account in his neighbourhood, but unless he could suddenly provide George with mobility, there was little chance of improvement. Finally, Neal asked one of Jack's harshest critics, Lynn Mills of Right to Life, to help George by linking him with a church or church group.

Lynn gave Neal the name of a Christian minister who visited George and subsequently assigned a parishioner to help him. The two developed a strong friendship. Later, when a prosecutor claimed that all of Kevorkian's patients ended up dead, George testified on Kevorkian's behalf.

George Murphy wasn't the only one Jack Kevorkian helped to live. Au Gres, Michigan is a small touristy town on Lake Huron about three hours' drive from Detroit. It is a beautiful place with up-scale shops and a marvellous shoreline. It is also a favourite retirement spot for the worn and weary from SE Michigan. Just south of Au Gres is a slightly larger town named Standish, a little more cosmopolitan in that it boasts the county hospital.

From Au Gres, the son of an elderly labour leader from Detroit petitioned Jack. The father was in his eighties and was suffering from congestive heart failure. He was the patriarch of a family of two sons and two daughters.

He was absolutely delighted to meet Dr Kevorkian, the renowned doctor who drove all the way to Au Gres just to meet with him. He hadn't spoken to such a notary since his early union days when he knew both Walter Reuther of the United

Auto Workers and Jimmy Hoffa of the Teamsters. He and Jack hit it off very well and enjoyed talk of the good old days when 'what was good for GM was good for America'.

He complained of pain, leg ulcerations caused by poor circu-lation and a desire to just end it all. When Jack asked the gentleman if he wanted to die, the answer was not a definitive 'yes'. It seemed that if it wasn't for his heart condition, he would want to go on living. Jack asked what the doctor had recommended, and was told he wanted to perform open-heart surgery at the local hospital.

While Standish General may have been a good hospital, Jack felt it wasn't the right place for this kind of operation. He had Neal set up an appointment with a specialist at St John's in Detroit, a leading hospital in major open-heart surgery at the time.

The old labourite did get his appointment at St John's but ulti-mately decided against an operation. His family doctor promised he would get good care in the Standish hospital and there he went. Neal Nicol visited a few weeks later and the old gentleman said he was still in pain so Neal complained to the only nurse he could find. She was on her coffee break but she said she would remedy the situation, albeit after her coffee was consumed. Neal related the story to one of the sons, who then got the family doctor to assure more palliative care. Although the old unionist did not live very much longer, his family had the relief of knowing that, with Jack's help, they were able to make the most informed medical decisions and bring their father to his natural end in as much comfort as possible and on their own terms.

There are other stories as well — stories of the loved ones of the deceased left behind to deal not only with their loss and grief, but in most cases having to deal with the attendant publicity and loss of privacy that occurred after Dr Kevorkian's participation was revealed.

Hugh Gale, for instance, an emphysema sufferer, decided he had had enough of life and told his wife Cheryl that all he wanted for Christmas was a visit from Jack Kevorkian. After his death no one gave a second thought to the life of his loved ones. Cheryl Gale was left alone in a house surrounded by crime scene tape, hounded by ubiquitous reporters, her neighbours badgered by the police. When the uproar died down, Cheryl, 46, was still alone with her memories, and had few to talk to about her loss and the method of her loss. Hugh had five grown sons by a previous marriage, but Cheryl had only her mother close by. Death is incomprehensible enough for survivors under 'normal' circumstances, but under these abnormal conditions it is still more difficult.

Jack decided that his patients' family members should meet, and Neal, Margo, her daughter Ava and Jack hosted a dinner for half a dozen survivors.

Many lasting friendships were initiated that day. Finally the bereaved had people with whom they could talk openly about the threats and recriminations of the press and police, as well as their respective losses. Calling themselves 'The Survivors', they often assisted other families through the difficult times following a medicide. They also walked picket lines and worked petition drives. Once, while picketing the Oakland County Jail where Jack was on a hunger strike, a minister showed up dressed like a high plains drifter, carrying a large photograph of Jack with a Hitler moustache painted on his face and shouting, 'Christians unite, Christians beware, Murderer.' This prompted the picket line to begin chanting 'Christians for Jack. Christians for Jack.' Doreen Ackner chanted 'Jews for Jack.' This was a group of ordinary people under very unordinary, stressful circumstances.

In 1995, Jack Lessenberry wrote in the Oakland Press:

> They are the forgotten people in the bitter dispute over assisted suicide, the ones left to cope with grief and stress while attracting little notice, even from those passionately for or against Dr Jack Kevorkian.
>
> They call themselves 'the survivors' – the family members and close friends of the people who have committed suicide with Kevorkian's help. Some say the police have harassed them. Many complain of being badgered by the media. A few have been forced to testify in criminal trials, and one was threatened with prosecution. Quietly, without fanfare and away from the media, they meet several times a year, over barbecues and potluck suppers, to offer support to each other.
>
> In 1995 more than a dozen survivors crowded into Neal Nicol's ranch house to chat with each other and with the man they regard as a hero, Jack Kevorkian. 'Whatever anyone else says, for us he'll always be a saint,' said Doreen Ackner, whose sister, Elaine Goldbaum, died in February 1993.

As difficult as it is for survivors to cope with their loss, they do have the comfort of knowing that they helped their loved one end their suffering and find the peace they were seeking. This was much less difficult than watching a family member live through horrible pain and debilitating illness. One son, who asked that his and his family's name not be used, described his mother's painful decline:

Mother was about 47 when she developed rheumatoid arthritis and her circulatory system went out of whack. During the next 22 years she not only suffered excruciating pain, but also seven unsuccessful operations.

The first catastrophic operation was to again correct Mother's eyesight (she previously had seven cornea transplants which were in addition to the above-mentioned operations). Blood wasn't circulating to her cornea, it ulcerated and she was in terrific pain. The hospital staff put a compact over the ulcer and ignored Mother's screams. Yet the next day the eye 'exploded' and it had to be removed. The operation was deemed a success by the medical staff.

The next operation was an attempt to un-mangle her gnarled hands. At this stage of her disease, mother could only use one finger to tap the telephone pad. The doctors slit open the backs of all her fingers enabling tendon transplants. Aspirin was the painkiller of choice offered in these early stages of her deterioration. The operation was a 'success', but the distortion soon recurred and left her with two fists and one free finger.

Mother developed pneumonia and had to be hospitalised. This short visit lasted seven weeks because while there they amputated her left leg just below the knee. Then, handling her after the operation, they broke her hip. That's when this sweet, alert, mentally sound woman entreated her sons to contact Dr Kevorkian.

We weren't ready to accept the inevitable, and Dad feared the reporters would turn the event into a freak show. But Mother was strong, forceful and wilful. We sent a video Mother made to Geoffrey Fieger and a session was scheduled with Dr Kevorkian for September 20th, 1992.

At the meeting all three of us boys were there, Mother, Dad, Neal Nicol, Dr Kevorkian and his sister Margo. Dr Kevorkian immediately put our minds at ease. He opened the session by telling us that this was just an open and frank discussion and nothing was binding. He asked questions about our families, our upbringing, our religion, our thoughts about Mother and Dad, and our feelings about losing Mother.

Dr Kevorkian stated that Mother might still have some worthwhile, although certainly not quality, time left. Dad could still tend to her, have the grandchildren visit, and her medication could still control her pain to some degree. What he offered more than anything was relief from fear and panic because if things got substantially worse, she could always call him again.

Over the next two years, Mother's pain increased and circulation and mobility decreased. The one 'good' leg wasn't doing too well and, as expected, it was amputated as well, this time above the knee. Mother by this time was obviously confined to a wheelchair and Dad, stalwart as ever, made the meals and fed her, carried her to and from bed, on and off the potty, and cleaned everything. The family couldn't afford an attending nurse but Dad didn't complain.

Mother's only real joy was when her grandchildren visited and she could watch them, barely, play in the kitchen and back yard. The doctor prescribed four Darvocet tablets a day that she hoarded for evening so she could at least sleep at night. But the pain was constant. Mother went on until March 1994 when the pain was so intense that we again called Dr Kevorkian. The surgical specialist wouldn't prescribe either a morphine patch or pump unless she was hospitalised; he wouldn't prescribe stronger painkillers to an outpatient. With her history, it's easy to appreciate Mother's reluctance to go back into a hospital.

We decided to produce an anonymous video, one from the neck down, which captured Mother's plight, and then distribute it to local television stations. The video was picked up nationwide. There was an outflow of disbelief and passion. Several doctors offered to control her pain and suffering by administering morphine. Her family physician claimed he was unaware of her strife and was now embarrassed into prescribing the drug.

Mother got some relief at last.

Regrettably, her relief only lasted until November when the morphine started to become ineffective. Mother again asked to see Dr Kevorkian.

At this point, we were 100 per cent behind Mother's decision. She had talked to her pastor, her family physician and her friends. They advised her to bear with it. As Mother said, 'They're not the ones to bear it.' She was asked if she was afraid to die and responded that she was afraid to live. The procedure was explained to both Mother and Dad as to how she had to initiate the process herself with her one 'good' finger. She was then asked two final questions: 'Have you changed your mind? Is there anything we can do to change your mind?' She said her only fear was that she would reawaken. Neal Nicol assured her that they had yet to save a patient. Neal held her hand and she went very peacefully.

This woman and her family might not have had to go through years of suffering were it not for America's archaic approach to drug control. Although the field of pain management has expanded and improved in recent years, there are still layers of bureaucratic stubbornness that make prescribing drugs for those who truly need them cumbersome – if not downright impossible. The medical establishment has a great fear that patients – even terminally ill patients – will become addicted to these drugs. However, no one has yet proven that pain management leads to drug abuse or addiction.

State panels monitor the number of prescriptions a doctor writes for controlled substances like morphine. If they deem that a doctor has written too many of these prescriptions, the doctor could very well lose his or her licence.

And if someone like Jack Kevorkian tries to change the laws in America so that those who can no longer manage their pain can die with dignity, he could very well lose his freedom. If it was up to Oakland County Prosecutor's office Jack would have been in jail soon after he assisted Janet Adkins. The prosecutor's frustration continued to grow as the state of Michigan, and the entire country, grappled with the medical, ethical and legal situation Dr Jack Kevorkian was forcing them to face.

Chapter 10

TRIALS AND ERRORS

In the introduction to her book, *Current Controversies: Assisted Suicide,* editor Laura K Egendorf wrote:

> He may be its most recognised practitioner, but Jack Kevorkian did not invent assisted suicide ... In ancient Greece, the government gave hemlock to those who wanted it. William Shakespeare memorialised the Roman practice in *Julius Caesar* by depicting Brutus running into the sword held by Strato. Opposition to the practice is also not new, including in the United States; by 1868, more than half of the thirty-seven states in the nation prohibited assisted suicide.

The opposition to assisted suicide, as Jack Kevorkian found out, continued into modern times. Between the years of 1990 and 1998, Jack Kevorkian spent almost as much time fighting the authorities as he did performing his medicides.

Before the legal system tried to stop his activities, the medical community did what it could. In 1991, his licence to practise medicine in Michigan was suspended. In 1993, his California licence was suspended because, according to that state's attorney general, Kevorkian was 'fundamentally unfit to practise medicine'.

Once the legal system started after Jack, prosecutors were determined to see him behind bars. Little did they know they would have to go through three acquittals and a mistrial to get him there. This timeline shows the many twists and turns along the way:

June 4th, 1990: Janet Adkins' assisted suicide.

December 13th, 1990: Murder charge that had been brought against Kevorkian for Adkins' death is dropped when a state judge rules Michigan has no law against assisted suicide.

October 23rd, 1991: Wantz and Miller medicides are performed.

February 28th, 1992: Kevorkian is charged with murders of Wantz and Miller.

July 21st, 1992: State judge dismisses Wantz and Miller murder charges, again because of no law against assisted suicide.

December 15th, 1992: Michigan governor John Engler signs temporary ban on assisted suicide.

August 4th, 1993: Thomas Hyde medicide is performed.

September 10th, 1993: Kevorkian is charged with murder of Thomas Hyde. That night, he performs assisted suicide of Donald O'Keefe, a 73-year-old man suffering from bone cancer.

September 11th, 1993: Kevorkian charged with murder of Donald O'Keefe.

November 22nd, 1993: Merian Frederick and Dr Ali Khalili medicides.

November 29th, 1993: Kevorkian charged in Frederick's death. He refuses to pay bond, goes to jail and goes on a hunger strike.

December 14th, 1993: Charges dropped in O'Keefe case when a judge rules assisted suicide law unconstitutional. Another judge, however, orders Kevorkian to stand trial for Frederick's death.

December 17th, 1993: Bond is posted, Kevorkian leaves jail. (The bond was paid by a Maryland tax assessor who vowed that if Jack died in jail he would commit suicide.)

January 4th, 1994: Kevorkian charged in Khalili's death.

January 27th, 1994: Circuit Judge Jessica Cooper dismisses assisted suicide charges against Kevorkian in the Frederick and Khalili cases.

May 2nd, 1994: Kevorkian acquitted in Hyde case.

May 10th, 1994: Michigan Court of Appeals orders murder charges reinstated in Wantz and Miller cases. Court also says assisted suicide law invalid on technical grounds.

December 13th, 1994: Michigan Supreme Court rules assisted suicide law is constitutional.

April 24th, 1995: US Supreme Court declines to hear appeals of Michigan Supreme Court ruling.

August 31st, 1995: Noting State Supreme Court ruling, Cooper sets trial date in Frederick and Khalili cases.

February 20th, 1996: Trial begins in Frederick and Khalili cases.

March 8th, 1996: Kevorkian acquitted in deaths of Frederick and Khalili.

April 16th, 1996: Trial begins in Oakland County on common-law assisted suicide charges in the deaths of Miller and Wantz.

May 14th, 1996: Jury acquits Kevorkian in deaths of Miller and Wantz.

August 30th, 1996: Loretta Peabody's assisted suicide.

November 8th, 1996: Kevorkian charged with murder of Loretta Peabody.

June 12th, 1997: Kevorkian goes on trial for death of Loretta Peabody. A mistrial is declared and Kevorkian is not retried for this death.

September 17th, 1998: Thomas Youk's assisted suicide.

November 22nd, 1998: *60 Minutes* shows tape of Kevorkian giving lethal injection to Thomas Youk.

November 28th, 1998: Kevorkian is charged with first-degree murder, violating the assisted suicide law and delivering a controlled substance in the death of Thomas Youk.

March 26th, 1999: Kevorkian convicted of a lesser charge of second-degree murder for the death of Thomas Youk.

Many Michigan prosecutors wanted to – tried to – bring charges against Jack, but were stopped by the fact that the state had no law against assisted suicide. A typical example is the case of Hugh Gale, the 70-year-old emphysema sufferer who Jack assisted in February 1993. Macomb County Prosecuting Attorney Carl J Marlinga came to a decision that Jack could not be charged, and stated his reasons in a memorandum dated April 27th, 1993:

DECISION

It is my decision that no charges will be filed against Dr Jack Kevorkian or any other person in connection with the death of Hugh Gale. Mr Gale's death can only be regarded as a suicide. Those present at the time of his death did nothing more than provide the means for him to accomplish a result that he desired. The great weight of evidence is that he never faltered in that desire up to the point that he lost consciousness.

REASONS FOR DECISION

At the time of Hugh Gale's death there was no law in Michigan making it a crime for a person to assist another in committing suicide. Case law was divided on the question of whether murder statutes could be expanded to apply to an assisted suicide case. In *People* v *Roberts*, 211 Mich 187, 178 NW 2d 690 (1920), the furnishing of poison by a husband to his invalid wife was held to be first degree murder. (The authority of the case is weakened, however, by the fact that the defendant pled guilty, thereby conceding the propriety of the conviction and arguing only the degree of murder on appeal.)

In August 1993, Jack Kevorkian became the first person charged under Michigan's new law banning assisted suicide. It was a felony that carried a penalty of up to four years in prison. Wayne County Prosecutor John D O'Hair was actually reluctant to charge Jack with the death of Thomas Hyde, but Kevorkian and Geoffrey Fieger pushed the issue: shortly after the death of Thomas Hyde, Jack acknowledged breaking the law and dared the prosecutor to charge him.

According to an August 18th, 1993 article in the *New York Times,* Mr O'Hair 'hoped a trial would encourage the courts and the State Legislature to move more quickly in resolving the issue of assisted suicide ... Whatever one's opinion of Dr Kevorkian is, he has nevertheless focused public attention and concern on this critical issue. He has served a useful purpose.'

The trial took place in May 1994. In his opening argument, Geoffrey Fieger stated:

> humanity and compassion are on trial. You will be deciding one of the great issues in the struggle for human rights ... His intent is never to kill someone, but only to reduce suffering. That is Dr Jack Kevorkian. That is the man who stands charged before you. You will decide how much suffering all of us must endure before we go into that good night – some of us, not so gently.

Jack Lessenberry wrote in a July 1994 article for *Vanity Fair* that:

> Jack heard little of the oration. To him, it is all a farce and a game. 'I am only going along with it to make Geoffrey feel good,' he whispered ... While Fieger thundered, trying to set the stage for a decision as momentous as *Roe* v. *Wade,* his client ... intently studied vocabulary lists of Japanese verbs.

During the trial, Fieger played the consultation tape Kevorkian had made of Hyde asking to die. Many of the jurors cried as they watched. On May 2nd, 1994, the jury found Jack Kevorkian not guilty of all charges.

Two years later, in February 1996, Jack was again on trial – this time for the deaths of Merian Frederick and Dr Ali Khalili. The problem for prosecutors in this trial was that the law against assisted suicide had been so quickly enacted and so poorly worded that it included several loopholes. In part, it read 'a person is not guilty of criminal assistance of suicide if that person was administering medications or procedures with the intent to relieve pain and discomfort and not to cause death', even if the treatment 'may hasten or increase the risk of death'.

Throughout the trial, Kevorkian repeatedly said that he did not want Frederick or Khalili to die, but that their deaths were an 'unfortunate, repugnant, unavoidable' consequence of relieving their pain and discomfort.

Prosecutor John Skrzynski tried to paint Kevorkian as an out-of-control mad scientist; the jury was not persuaded. They were, instead, sympathetic when Geoffrey Fieger produced friends and family of the deceased who testified that the patients had been suffering horribly and had sought help from Dr Kevorkian. On March 8th, 1996, the not-guilty verdicts were read by the jury foreman, the Rev Donald Ott, a Methodist bishop.

At a press conference following the verdict, Jack stated:

> This is not a personal victory for me. I give you my oath that if I ever am involved in this right of assisted suicide for a patient, for you, for anybody, I will not abuse it. And anything I do in connection with it will always be for human welfare and for human benefit. Always, no matter how distasteful or repugnant it may seem to some.

Defeated by the vagaries of their own law (which was temporary and had expired in November 1994), prosecutors took a different tack in the April 1996 trial for the deaths of Marjorie Wantz and Sherry Miller. Originally, prosecutor Richard Thompson had

sought to charge Kevorkian with murder, but Oakland County
Circuit Court Judge David Breck dismissed the cases on the by
now familiar grounds that Michigan had no law against assisted
suicide. However, in December 1994, the Michigan Supreme
Court ruled that assisted suicide had always been a 'common-law
crime', meaning one that was based on custom rather than legislation. The statute reads:

> Any person who shall commit any indictable offence at the
> common law for the punishment of which no provision is
> expressly made by any statute of this State shall be guilty of
> a felony punishable by imprisonment in the State prison not
> more than five years or by a fine of not more than $10,000.00
> or both at the discretion of the court.

Attorney Michael Schwartz explained in 1995, after Jack had been
charged with the deaths of Wantz and Miller:

> This essentially says if Michigan legislation did not think
> that they wanted to make a law saying something was
> criminal, or if it was something that which in the old
> days in Jolly Olde England would have been a crime
> under common law, then the five-year felony would apply.
> Assisting in suicide is a common law, as is suicide itself, but it
> is very difficult to try the latter because the purported felon
> is dead. Most of American civil law is based on the common
> law. Criminal law is rarely based on common law because
> in the United States criminal law is codified, enacted by
> legislation.

The case was reopened and Kevorkian went to trial in May 1996.

For the start of the trial, Jack wore a colonial costume – tights, a powdered wig and big buckle shoes – to protest the fact that he was being tried under a centuries-old law. During the trial, the prosecutor asked:

> Prosecutor: How do you determine before you'll agree to help, for example, Marjorie Wantz, that she'd suffered enough?
>
> Kevorkian: Given enough time, you see if there's any ret-rogression of the process or any progression or any kind of amelioration. It's subjective. Many medical diagnoses and interpretations are subjective. That's why this can't be legis-lated.
>
> Prosecutor: You are aware that three psychiatrists in Michi-gan had determined that Marjorie Wantz was mentally ill and needed psychiatric treatment, is that correct?
>
> Kevorkian: Yes, and I was aware of others who said she wasn't. It was a split opinion. I was aware of a split opinion. Don't make it sound like it's one way.
>
> Prosecutor: Oh, if you got three psychiatrists that say she is in need of mental health treatment, but two other ones that say she's not, you're the umpire? You can say, 'Touchdown. She can die'?
>
> Kevorkian: I knew she was sane, so if it's a split decision, I rely on my good judgment. Even though I'm not a psychiatrist, I can judge an insane person pretty well.

Fieger's defence of Jack was mainly based on the fact that there had never been a prior case of using common law to prosecute assisted suicide. At one point, Jack shouted from the witness stand, 'There ain't no law. I only recognise laws passed by a legislature, not made up by courts.'

In a May 15th, 1996 *New York Times* article, the jury, which came back with a not-guilty verdict, indicated that:

> those arguments had been telling. One of them, Mary Hess, 59, a technical worker for a suburban school system, said she initially believed the doctor was guilty. But over the weekend, Ms Hess said, as she was raking leaves in her back yard, 'I realised I didn't want someone to come along three years from now and say that raking leaves back then was illegal, you just didn't know it.'

'The juries saw the condition the deceased were in,' said Michael Schwartz after the trial:

> and everyone could relate to someone, a mother, an uncle, a brother, a friend, a neighbour, that had a horrible, horrible fateful disease. Cancer, Alzheimer's, Lou Gehrig's Disease – diseases that ravaged their hosts, diseases that literally tortured them to death because there aren't any cures for these misfortunes and the end is just the same. People can understand how someone suffering such affliction may not want to go on, go through the torture. They understand it's their choice, their right, and anyone assisting them is doing them a favour and shouldn't be punished for this humanitarian act.

The June 1997 trial for the death of Loretta Peabody was the shortest one for Kevorkian. In September 1996, Royal Oak police raided a meeting between Kevorkian and a Fresno, California woman who was seeking Jack's help. During that raid, police discovered a videotaped conference between Jack and Loretta Peabody, taped in her kitchen the day she died. Iona County Prosecutor Raymond Voet and old adversary Oakland Country Prosecutor Richard Thompson decided to bring charges, despite the fact that Peabody's husband and daughter, subpoenaed to testify before the grand jury, decline to cooperate.

The case went to trial on June 13th, but was over shortly after it began. The judge declared a mistrial after Geoffrey Fieger, in his opening statement, accused the prosecutor of harassing witnesses and altering evidence. Judge Charles Miel said that Fieger's remarks were prejudicial and that the impartiality of some jurors might be affected.

After the trial, Ray Voet said, 'That was the most outrageous, illegal opening statement I've seen in my life.' Geoffrey Fieger, on the other hand, stated that he thought Mr Voet had 'ended the case precipitously, because he knew what I was going to do to him'. The prosecutors decided not to retry the case.

Jack was not tried again until March 1999, when he was convicted for the death of Thomas Youk.

Of course, not everyone agreed with the jurors in the Kevorkian acquittals. Many of the disabled and their advocates saw Jack's efforts as attempts to 'cleanse' society of people like themselves. Several times, vans full of the disabled would arrive at the courthouse where they would disembark and lie down in the road or on the courthouse steps, unable to move, while their able-bodied advocates shouted through bullhorns, 'Hey, hey, ho, ho, Doctor Death has got to go.'

Numerous times, Right-to-Lifers would congregate at court, outside Jack's home or at any venue where he or the press were present, or expected to be present, and shout 'Kill Kevorkian' over and over again.

Attorney Michael Schwartz may have said it best:

> It's sad when Jack is trying to accomplish something, with the vast majority, over 80 per cent, in his corner and religious and political people, the political system, can side-step it, violate it; it's unbelievable. It's like the abortion situation. Whether you believe in it or not, I can't comprehend someone saying to another individual, 'I believe that life is sacred and if you commit abortion I'll kill you.' It's the same with Jack. I can't see the logic of these people saying what they say about assisted suicide. The Right-to-Lifers have no compassion for people in desperate straits and want to either destroy Jack or have him killed. It's beyond my comprehension that there are people believing in the sacredness of life and yet who are ready and willing to kill.

Against this backdrop, Jack and his supporters made several attempts to promote and legalise assisted suicide in Michigan. Jack initiated the first attempt in June 1994. Margo and Neal Nicol went to Lansing to drop off the proposed wording on the petition and get the state's permission to circulate it in an effort to get it on the ballot and allow the people of Michigan to vote on the issue. Margo and Jack set up an office and began contacting churches and right-to-die groups for support.

The actual wording on the petition was:

A petition to amend Article 1 of the Michigan constitution, by adding a section 25, which would read as follows: THE RIGHT OF COMPETENT ADULTS, WHO ARE INCAPACITATED BY INCURABLE MEDICAL CONDITIONS, TO VOLUNTARILY REQUEST AND RECEIVE MEDICAL ASSISTANCE WITH RESPECT TO WHETHER OR NOT THEIR LIVES CONTINUE, SHALL NOT BE RESTRAINED OR ABRIDGED.

This was known as the MERCY campaign (Movement to Ensure the Right to Choose for Yourself). It was at this time that Janet Good and volunteers from the Hemlock Society of Michigan became involved with Jack. The abbreviated wording of the petition allowed the issue to be easily explained. Jack, Margo, Neal and other volunteers attempted to collect the needed 256,457 valid signatures within 180 days of the first signature, as required. They collected 175,000, and paid solicitors and newspaper ballots collected another 30,000 by the deadline, but as they fell short by over 50,000 signatures the question wasn't put on the ballot.

In 1995, a small group of doctors calling themselves Physicians for Mercy offered their public support to Dr Kevorkian. This was the first time he had received any organised support from the medical community. The physicians included nephrologists Dr Mohammed El Nachef, psychologist Dr Stephen Hnat, psychiatrist Dr William Kimbrough, internist Dr Stan Levy (presently Dr Kevorkian's personal physician), surgeon Dr Nicholas Renziparis and family practitioner Dr Roy Cooley.

They announced a set of guidelines they had approved for physician-assisted suicide, which included a written request dated, signed and notarised by the patient, a doctor and two witnesses having no financial relationship with the patient and examination by a specialist in the patient's specific illness, a pain specialist and a psychiatrist, to assure the patient's mental competence. The final procedure was to be performed by an obiatrist, a doctor specific to these procedures, within 72 hours of the signing of informed consent, but no sooner than 24 hours. There was to be no professional fee charged for the service. They helped Jack with one assisted suicide, but beyond their guidelines they did not make any great effort to change the law.

The second campaign to legalise assisted suicide in Michigan was headed by Dr Edward Pierce. It was called 'Merian's Friends' after Jack's patient, Merian Frederick. Her daughter Carol Poenish served as treasurer on the campaign. The campaign ran in 1998 and they had the same 180 days to collect 379,000 signatures to assure that their assisted-suicide initiative measure – entitled 'Terminally Ill Patient's Right to End Unbearable Pain or Suffering' (also known as Proposal B) – was eligible for placement on the state's November 3rd ballot. This campaign was much more efficiently organised than the first one, more funds were raised for advertising and for paid solicitors, and the group was able to gather enough voter signatures to qualify. But, on election day, Michigan voters handed assisted-suicide proponents an overwhelming defeat, rejecting Proposal B by a margin of 71 per cent to 29. Even Jack publicly stated that he would not vote for this law, because the petition had covered four sheets of small print and imposed too many restrictions. Many church groups were active in their opposition to the petition, and it was defeated.

Many mainstream churches, however, definitely and defiantly backed Kevorkian. Several Unitarian and Presbyterian churches in the greater Detroit area allowed petition campaign meetings to be held in their churches. Jack also assisted one male Unitarian minister, married to a female Unitarian minister, to end his pain. Many of the clergy preached favourably of assisted suicide from the pulpit.

In fact, most of America was, and is, in favour of some form of assisted suicide. Sixty-five per cent of those polled in June 1990 by *USA Today*, when Jack performed his first medicide, agreed that the terminally ill should be granted medical help to end their lives. The *United Methodist Reporter*, published in Dallas that same year, revealed that 73 per cent of its readers believe that it is morally justified for an individual to commit suicide under some circumstances. A February 1991 poll of *Longevity* magazine revealed that 86 per cent of those responding answered 'yes' when asked: 'is it ever proper for a doctor to assist a patient in committing suicide?' In a CNN/*USA Today* Gallup poll of 1,022 adults conducted during the first week of January 1997, 58 per cent said doctors should be allowed to help a terminally ill patient die if the patient is in severe pain and asks for assistance. Forty per cent said they would consider suicide themselves.

The Pew Research Center for The People and The Press found in a November 2005 survey, that 'while overall attitudes are largely stable, people are increasingly thinking about – and planning for – their own medical treatment in the event of a terminal illness or incapacitating medical condition'. It also found that 'the public is deeply divided over legalizing physician–assisted suicide; 46% approve of laws permitting doctors to help patients to end their lives, while about as many are opposed (45%)'. However, these views were greatly affected by the amount of thought given to end-of-life issues. According to the poll, '57% of those who have given a great deal of thought to these issues approve of legal assisted suicide, a view shared by only 35% of those who have given little or no thought to these matters.'

In one part of the United States, voters were taking more than polls. Janet Adkins was from Oregon, and her husband Ron spearheaded a movement that resulted, in a general election in November 1994, with the citizens of the state of Oregon passing the first and, so far, the only physician assisted suicide law in the country. It was won by a margin of 51 per cent to 49 per cent. An injunction was immediately placed against it, but was lifted in October of 1997, and in November of that year, a measure was placed on the general election ballot to repeal the Death with Dignity Act (as the law was called). Voters, by a margin of 60 per cent to 40 per cent, chose to retain the act. In 2006, justices at the US Supreme Court voted 6–3 to uphold the law, under which doctors are thought to have assisted with at least 208 suicides. According to the BBC, three of the judges had had cancer, and one had a wife who counsels dying young cancer patients.

The Death with Dignity Act permits physicians to write prescriptions for a lethal dosage of medication to people with a terminal illness. The law states that, in order to participate, a patient must be:

1. 18 years of age or older;
2. a resident of Oregon;
3. capable of making and communicating health care decisions for him/herself; and
4. diagnosed with a terminal illness that will lead to death within six months.

Two doctors must agree that the patient is mentally competent and that the decision was voluntary. The law does not require that the physician be present when the patient takes lethal medication. A physician may be present if a patient wishes it, as long as the physician does not administer the medication him or herself.

There are only three other places that legally authorise active assistance in dying of patients. Switzerland passed a law in 1941 authorising physician and non-physician assisted suicide only, but not euthanasia; in 2002 Belgium permitted 'euthanasia' but did not define the method; and in the Netherlands voluntary euthanasia and physician-assisted suicide have been lawful since April 2002, but have been permitted by the courts since 1984.

In Canada, both assisted suicide and euthanasia or mercy killing are illegal. The Canadian Criminal Code states, 'Anyone who helps or counsels a person to commit suicide could go to jail. No one can take the life of another, even in mercy, or even at the request of the person.'

Sue Rodriguez, a young mother from British Columbia with Lou Gehrig's disease, was the first person to challenge Canada's law. From 1992 to 1994, Canadians supported this brave woman as she publicly battled both her disease and the courts in the media. On September 29th, 1993, Sue Rodriguez lost her legal fight. The Supreme Court, in a marginal 5–4 decision, ruled that an individual's right to a dignified death does not override the sanctity of life under the law. Sue defied the law against doctor-assisted suicide and on February 12th, 1994 took her life, presumably with the help of drugs administered by an unidentified physician.

There have been many public debates following Sue's demise, but the law hasn't changed. One positive result was that it brought the debate on the subject into the open. Another positive outcome has been the legalisation of marijuana for severe pain sufferers. This is controlled by a government agency, similar to the FDA, allowing the purchase of quality controlled substances. Unfortunately, only small amounts are meted out, and when the power of the drug has elapsed, there is no recourse but to suffer in silence.

Due to the court's decision, Austin Bastable of Windsor, Ontario, a former tool and die maker, came to the US for the assistance of Dr Kevorkian. With the exception of minor mobility in one arm, multiple sclerosis had paralysed him from the neck down. He was confined to a bed where his only motor ability was to lift and lower himself by a bar hung above the bed. His working wife, Nina, had to feed him, wash him and provide toilet availability. He cancelled his beloved *National Geographic* because he couldn't even turn a page. When asked his favourite time of day, Austin said when sleeping because once he is lifted into bed and falls asleep, that day's struggle had ended.

In 1994, prior to his total incapacity, he wheeled himself into his kitchen, drank a couple of Rob Roys with a bunch of sleeping pills and tried to die. Nina came home from work and found him slumped in his wheelchair with his chin on his chest, saw the bottles, panicked and called 911. When he awoke in the hospital 36 hours later, Nina apologised for her interference.

Austin then decided he would go on for a few years to not only fight his disease but to wrestle with the Canadian government in an attempt to have Parliament change its medieval laws on assisted suicide. He collected 2,500 petition signatures, opened a website called 'S-O-S: Message from a Dying Man' and sent letters to Canadian Parliament members in an effort to force a vote on the issue. They had no effect.

Austin dictated his eulogy and he recorded a videotape to be played to the press after he died. He even requested the undertaker's makeup artist to mould a smile on his face to convey that he was happy to be dead. He believed that death was 'just another step' that brings something he didn't have, peace. In the spring of 1996, after the usual prerequisites demanded by Jack, Austin was delivered by his wife to Jack via the Detroit–Windsor tunnel and US Customs. He was driven to a private home in Farmington, MI where he met Jack, Neal, Janet Good, her husband Ray and the supportive doctors of the Physicians for Mercy.

In his videotaped consultation, Austin is heard bantering, joking and laughing. One of the doctors says, 'I think you're saner than I am.' Austin, growing tired of Jack's repeated questions: 'Do you really want to die? Are you sure?' answered, 'You know, boys, it's getting kind of late. I'm pretty pooped. Let's get on with it.'

After a private talk with Nina, Austin started the suicide machine.

Nina returned to Canada, through Canadian Customs, to a funeral home. As in the US, the police and press had a field day. Canadian authorities threatened to extradite Jack to stand trial. They threatened Nina with assisted suicide, smuggling and other border violations and effectively frightened her out of continuing Austin's crusade against the government. There was, however, a very large right-to-die contingent at Austin's funeral, and the authorities eventually dropped their harassment and threats in fear of escalating the argument for assisted suicide and losing a lawsuit, thus creating a larger problem for themselves.

There have been other high-profile cases since. None have changed the law, despite a 1997 poll taken by Canadian polling firm Pollara that found that 70 per cent of Canadians said assisted suicide was allowable in some circumstances and that 60 per cent were in favour of legalising it.

In England and Wales, assisted suicide is illegal and punishable by up to 14 years imprisonment. Between 1936 and 2003, eight different bills or amendments were introduced into Parliament to allow carefully monitored physician-assisted suicide, but none succeeded. However, the Dignitas clinic in Switzerland has helped over 40 people from the UK to legally die. Dr Anne Turner, 66, had a progressive and incurable degenerative disease called supranuclear palsy, and had already seen her husband and brother suffer lingering deaths. With the charities help, she committed suicide in Switzerland on January 24th, 2006. Before she left the UK she said:

> Doctors should be able to help people to die. I always quote the fact that I had a cat, and I had him put down because he was riddled with cancer, but we cannot do that with humans at all now ...
>
> I feel strongly that assisted suicide should become legal in this country. In order to ensure that I am able to swallow the medication that will kill me, I have to go to Switzerland before I am totally incapacitated and unable to travel.
>
> If I knew that when things got so bad, I would be able to request assisted suicide in Britain, then I would not have to die before I am completely ready to do so.

A law to make physician-assisted suicide illegal is due to be considered in the House of Lords. Assisted suicide is a crime in Ireland. In Scotland, suicide is not a crime, and the courts have never tested whether it is criminal to help someone commit suicide; however, a person could be brought up on charges such as recklessly endangering human life.

In Australia, which has a strong right-to-die movement, voluntary euthanasia and assisted suicide were legalised in the Northern Territory in 1997. However, the law was repealed seven months later by the Federal Parliament. In January 2006, the Criminal Code Amendment (Suicide Related Material Offences) Act 2005 went into effect, which prohibits the transmission of information about methods of suicide by email, internet, fax or phone. Individuals who break the law are subject to a A$120,000 fine, and organisations could be hit with a fine of A$500,000.

Chapter 11

ECCENTRICITIES

Against this backdrop of controversy around the world, Jack remained an eccentric character, amusing and exasperating his closest associates in equal amounts. He spent much of his time concerned about the petty details of life. One of his most constant concerns was his 'trusty' VW van, which Jack used to assist his patients, and frequently to deliver them to the coroner's office. Old and rusty, there were no carpets, power brakes or power steering. Jack was inordinately proud of the side rearview mirrors, which he had crafted himself out of aluminium, hammering each piece around a glass mirror.

Neal remembers travelling to the coroner's office late one night. Jack was to drop off his deceased patient in the van and then join Neal in his car for the trip home. It was around midnight, and as Neal was driving along he saw Jack suddenly pull into the side of the road. Neal continued along for another block or so and waited at the next light to see if Jack was following. He waited for some time, and then, thinking the van had a breakdown, turned around and drove back and found Jack still parked at the side of the road. Jack said, 'Oh,

I had to take off my mirrors, you know the darn cops might steal them.'

Neal thought this hilarious. Jack was delivering a body at midnight to the coroner's office knowing full well that all hell would break loose, and there he was worrying about his homemade, worthless mirrors.

Jack hated taking bodies to coroners' offices because his van was always confiscated. The police would keep it for two or three days until they were satisfied that it was well dusted for prints and, with lawyer inducement, release it. They were probably keeping the van just to irritate him, and in this endeavour they were exceedingly successful as Jack fumed and stewed, ranted and raved. He would call them day in, day out to get the release, haranguing his lawyers, the prosecuting attorneys and cops alike, and generally work himself into a lather. Every time Jack used the van to drop off patients, the police dusted it for fingerprints. No matter how mottled it became with the black dust, Jack refused to wash it. It remained covered with dust until its eventual demise.

He went to pick up the van after one event and for some reason they gave it back without the licence plates. It was probably just another way of harassing him, as he could get pulled over and arrested for not having plates. Jack made up a sign that he displayed in the rear window that read, 'Sheriff Nicols Stole My License Plate!' He rode around town with that sign for several weeks, yet no one pulled him over.

A favourite recollection of Geoffrey Fieger's took place one summer night. Jack had asked Michael Schwartz and Fieger to meet him at Pontiac General Hospital, as an event was about to occur. They parked their car near the emergency entrance and were sitting there waiting for Jack to arrive. It was very dark and a light fog was swirling about the hospital because it was still 70 degrees Fahrenheit. They didn't see or hear Jack but a squeaky noise got their attention. Then, through the fog, the spectral form of Jack appeared pushing a deceased patient in a wheelchair as unconcerned as if he was on a stroll through Central Park. Jack wheeled the man through the emergency door, was inside for three or four minutes, and then nonchalantly returned. The eerie atmosphere, the squeak-squeak of the wheels and the emergence of Jack through the gloom pushing a cadaver is etched in Mike and Geoff's memories for ever.

Now that he was finally making a name for himself, being fully involved in challenging and significant work, Jack was able to take a step back, relax and make genuine friendships with other people. His very intimate work with the dying also gave him the ability to connect to the living. These were good days for Jack.

When he returned to Michigan from Los Angeles, Jack lived in a low-rent apartment on Main Street in Royal Oak, a trendy suburb of Detroit. His friends affectionately came to name the apartments the 'Kevorkian Arms Hotel'.

Kevorkian soon joined some fellow tenants for bi-monthly poker games. Jack's favourite game was straight five-card draw poker because it was not as cutthroat as some of the other forms. However, if the pot grew to more than two dollars Jack would drop out – that was too rich for his blood.

Neal Nicol recalls one game, following an arrest, in which Jack was on an electronic tether, a device that restricted his movements to his immediate environs. The apartment building had been recently condemned and was near razing, so Jack had acquired a vacant apartment in the building to hold the game – he didn't want to use his own because he didn't want gambling charges on top of his other problems. Neal remembers the empty apartment was like a set from a B movie – a bare kitchen with a bare light bulb hanging from the ceiling, a faucet dripping and outside wall cracks that made the flimsy curtains flutter in the wind. It was February and very cold. Jack had to sit closest to the door so as not to overextend his tether distance. All players were on edge, not from the stakes of the game but for fear of a raid.

That summer, when the building was actually being razed, the group held one last poker game in the Arms. One of the demolitionists crashed the party with an armload of bricks for Jack to sign as souvenirs. Jack accommodated him and then all the players received a signed brick as well. Even with all the paraphernalia garnered over the years with connection to Jack and his many avocations, Neal Nicol still treasures his autographed brick.

After the Kevorkian Arms was demolished, Jack moved to a small two-bedroom ranch-style house on a lake in West Bloomfield. The house, situated on a quiet dead end street, was owned by Geoffrey Fieger. Jack's new next-door neighbours were Harry and Arlene Wylie. Again, Jack was able to establish a good friendship with Harry, and soon Jack began bringing him to poker games, which now took place in the backroom of a bookstore.

Jack and his group of friends started playing golf before the card games, which eventually led to a foursome getting together about twice a week. The makeup of the group changed often – Jack and Neal were constant players, and they could be joined by Brian Russell, the owner of the bookstore, Michael Schwartz from Geoffrey Fieger's office, a couple of Neal's customers from his lab or sometimes just other golfers who were looking for players. Wearing K-Mart tennis shoes with overly long laces that he wrapped around his ankles and tied in big bows, for a while Jack became very enthusiastic about the game (until his lack of skill became too much for him). Jack favoured the course at Huntington Woods in Michigan – it had especially nice fruit trees and he hunted for apples and pears as often as his balls, which was often.

During every round, two or three players would approach Jack, shake his hand, and thank him for what he was doing. In one game a conversation developed around a condemned prisoner in Texas who wanted to donate his organs for transplantation. The state had denied his final attempt at societal restitution. Jack became upset over this matter and it was suggested he call Barbara Walters.

After they finished the round, the foursome went to the starter's shack where Jack pulled a small piece of paper from his wallet with *ABC News'* New York telephone number on it and proceeded to call Barbara. Barbara, however, had left for the day. Nonplussed, another piece of paper was extracted from the wallet and Jack phoned Barbara Walters at her home. His friends were amazed beyond words that this man, who they had played poker and golf with for years, had this national news figure's home number scrunched up in his wallet like a luncheon receipt and could simply call her up. Barbara raised the issue of the condemned man during a newscast a few days later. The boys thought it wonderful and astonishing that their friend had the notoriety and personality to talk to people of influence and get things done. To them he was just good old Jack.

At the end of the millennium, *Time* magazine held a gala event in New York City celebrating their 75th Jubilee. They invited all their 'cover stars', which included Jack. He and his date, one of Fieger's young female attorneys, Rebecca, were seated with Tom

Cruise and apparently he and Jack hit it off quite well. Rebecca was enamoured by Kevin Costner and asked Jack if he could introduce her to him. Kevin seemed to be continually preoccupied, however, so Jack yelled, 'Hey, Kevin, talk to this girl or I'll kill you!' Kevin did speak with Becky and Jack was quoted, with much amusement, the next day in the *New York Times*.

Jack continued to devise numerous incongruous business ideas. Despite poker and golf, sports were not one of Jack's favourite pastimes. He often remarked that Americans were more interested in Monday night football than current events, especially international events. This didn't stop him coming up with an idea for give-away visors at sport venues. He hand painted hundreds of cardboard visors for all the major sport teams in America. The Detroit Redwings' hats had floppy wings sailing away from the temples, the Minnesota Viking's visor had horns. The hats were colourful, inexpensive and, he thought, would be beautiful gifts for children. He tried to promote the idea to the Detroit Lions' front office, but when little interest was shown – because the team played indoors – Jack, in his usual fashion, lost interest in the project.

Harry Wylie was rather taken with the idea, and set up a meeting to display Jack's hats with the CEO of an international novelty gift company. A telemarketing conference was set up among their offices in Detroit, London, Toronto and New York and it seemed they were getting somewhere, but it turned out the CEO was more interested in meeting the infamous Dr Death than progressing the business idea.

Jack also devised a board game he called Cross-Mate that he envisioned worldwide participation and competition on the internet. The seed of the idea began germination when he was living in California, and was a combination of crossword puzzle and chess where the participants form increasingly difficult words to stump and eventually checkmate their opponent. Harry investigated several software designers on Jack's behalf, but the designers couldn't master the process for internet usage.

Back on the subject of assisted suicide, Jack published a book in 1991, *Prescription Medicide: The Goodness of Planned Death*, in which he explained his views on assisted suicide, and made his argument for organ donation from condemned prisoners. This book was aimed at the general public, but as with his published articles the response was sceptical. *Publisher's Weekly* called it a 'self-dramatizing, often strident manifesto'. Other publications saw its benefit as a research document, because it also included information about the modes of capital punishment through history; the *School Library Journal,* for instance, stated that it was 'valuable for students researching capital punishment'.

Jack also began painting again to promote and fund his crusade to legalise assisted suicide. They may not have helped his cause. Viewing them at an art show in 1997, Gretchen Voss wrote in *Boston Magazine* that 'They're more political cartoons than aesthetic masterpieces, the message of which chills your flesh ... [the paintings] offer a rare glimpse into the abyss of Jack Kevorkian's mind, and it's a pretty frightening place. As British psychologist Havelock Ellis wrote in his book *The New Spirit,* "every artist writes his own biography".' Some critics claimed that the disturbing images were a product of a sick mind, and therefore evidence that Jack engaged in assisted suicide not because of some noble inner calling, but because he was obsessed with death and enjoyed watching people die. However, there was also praise. Norbert Lakemaker, an artist at the Kastel Gallery, Montreal said:

> Art is a product of grief and suffering, the root of life is pain. Formally, painting was in the same line as literature, and was narrated. New art is drawing closer to music, as it is intended to have an effect on the emotions, in about the same manner as music which is, after all, also an abstract art. I believe that had Dr Kevorkian chosen to be an artist instead of being a doctor, he would have achieved even greater accomplishments. I appreciate his craftsmanship and skills in the same way as I do Dali. That said, his works make a statement to society that goes far beyond pleasing the human eye.

Jack had the most success with music. Music was, and still is, one of the most important aspects of his life. In 1997 he produced a jazz CD entitled *A Very Still Life*, in collaboration with The Morpheus Quintet. The CD reveals warm, musical and vulnerable aspects of his often misperceived personality. Jack improvises flute on eight out of nine of his compositions. One of his fellow musicians is quoted on the jacket:

> Every musician involved in the making of *A Very Still Life* has been surprised and motivated by the unexpected scope of Jack Kevorkian. His compositional efforts, represented here in irreverent new arrangements, have been inspirational – especially in light of the daily skirmishes he's compelled to wage on other far more fatiguing and treacherous fronts.

The CD was nominated for a Grammy Award in 1997.

In April 2000, Jack was awarded the Gleitsman Foundation Citizen Activist Award, which is designed to encourage individual commitment and leadership by recognising the exceptional achievement of people who have initiated social change. Bestowing the award on Kevorkian, Alan Gleitsman wrote:

> The efforts of Dr Kevorkian to confront, challenge and correct social injustice truly makes a difference in improving the quality of life in their communities. Throughout his career, Dr Kevorkian has been a selfless believer in death with dignity and has sacrificed his medical licence and now his freedom toward that cause.

Approximately 20 demonstrators opposed to assisted suicide – some of them with seeing-eye dogs and wheelchairs – protested the award ceremony. Jack had been in prison for more than a year by that time. The award was accepted on Jack's behalf by Thomas Youk's widow, Melody.

'He risked his personal freedom,' she said. 'Today he is in a very small cell, alone but not forgotten.'

In a letter read by his attorney, Kevorkian expressed gratitude for the award. The letter read: 'I certainly wish I could be there tonight, but in a real sense, I am. In spirit, I'm joining kindred souls in a ceremony celebrating the defense of a fundamental human liberty.'

Chapter 12

DEFENDING HIMSELF

Humanitarian awards aside, Dr Jack Kevorkian made many mistakes in his lifetime, as do we all, but his spate of errors on the road to Jackson Prison was without equal. His self-destruction was as precise and predictable as a class in anatomy:

1. Fire the lawyer who won every case the state levied against you.
2. Change your modus operandi, and
3. Brazenly parade yourself committing a probable crime on national television, to force the state into action.
4. Act as your own attorney at the trial of the century.
5. Hire two young, inexperienced attorneys to replace the indomitable firebrand.

All concerned forecast the outcome of his final conflict with the judiciary of Michigan. All, that is, except Jack.

His first error was the predictable rift between Jack and Geoffrey Fieger. Although asked many times, both erstwhile friends refuse to say what caused the estrangement. But causal evidence is apparent. They were best of friends, yet they were always at odds. They dined out together almost weekly and Jack was frequently invited to Geoffrey's home for dinner. They often went to movies together. Yet Jack's neighbour Harry Wylie recalls whenever he heard, from a considerable distance, Jack screaming on the phone, he knew he was probably talking with Fieger.

On one occasion Geoffrey told a Detroit TV audience that Jack was living in one of his houses pro bono. Jack ranted and raved to Harry that he was moving, to where he did not know, but he was getting out of there. He wasn't going to take Geoffrey's verbal abuse any longer. He was paying $235 a month rent to Geoffrey, and Geoffrey knew it. In reality, Geoffrey probably didn't know it. He almost certainly thought he was loaning the house to Jack at no cost. The payment would likely have gone directly to his law firm and Fieger would never have seen the transaction. Additionally, Geoffrey might have considered the $235 tantamount to pro bono. For a lakeside house in West Bloomfield, Michigan, it was next to nothing, but to Jack – whose income was based on his social security cheque, a retirement pension from Saratoga General Hospital, a few monetary awards and donations to his Penumbra Corporation – it was a *huge* amount of money.

The chief wedge driven between the two friends was probably Jack's insistence on representing himself at his trial. No lawyer worth his or her salt would to acquiesce to this foolishness.

Jack should have been, but wasn't, satisfied with the status quo he had achieved in Michigan. He could and did assist in helping the sick and dying, and assisted suicide was gaining acceptance. But other doctors hadn't come to the fore and openly assisted patients. There were no obitiatry clinics throughout the country. Jack wanted to get assisted suicide to the Supreme Court of the land and felt the only way this could happen was to get convicted. He was sure that he would never be found guilty as long as Geoffrey Fieger was his attorney.

Neal recalls an event, about the time of their separation, when Geoffrey and Jack had another yelling fest. Apparently Geoffrey promised *Time Life* magazine that a reporter could witness and photograph Jack's next assisted suicide. Jack nixed the idea pronouncing that the occasions were private moments for the families and should be treated with respect. Geoffrey retorted with vehemence, 'What's the matter with you? Can't you see the opportunity this would be for your cause? Someone's going to do it, and you're going to miss the opportunity!'

Journalist Jack Lessenberry wrote, generally favourably, about Kevorkian's trials for the *New York Times*, *Vanity Fair*, *Harpers* and other publications and became very well acquainted with Dr Kevorkian. He often went out on a limb for Jack and consequently endured a lot of criticism from readers and editors alike.

Lessenberry relates:

> A big part of the story people don't realise was Geoffrey Fieger and Jack Kevorkian were like father and son, except Fieger, who could have been Jack's son chronologically, acted more like the father, especially in legal matters. They would fight with one another, incessantly bicker, sometimes in public, but there was this quality of affection and respect. I think they delighted sometimes in driving one another nuts.
>
> On one occasion, Jack was in jail for three days, just released and Geoffrey had a piece of pie for Jack because he'd been on a hunger strike. Jack wrangled on as to what kind of pie it

was, how old, how much sugar and fat were in it, how bad it may be for his health, and on and on. 'Just eat the goddamn pie,' retorted Fieger.

They both needed one another, they both cared for one another a great deal and their self-imposed separation is indeed unfortunate. As long as the partnership worked, it was great. It enabled both of them to do what they do best and it's sort of tragic that the relationship came apart. They got on one another's nerves and Kevorkian, to be honest, has seldom or never been in a forum where he has not been the brightest person present. This has been the case all his life. This is not an ego trip on his part, but he has developed the sense that he can do anything. What he discovered he couldn't do was to act as his own lawyer.

Jack's second mistake was upping the odds, changing his modus operandi and administering euthanasia.

Jack Lessenberry commented:

> Jack became very frustrated with the legal system. They would go into one court and prove his innocence, then again, and another. It was déjà vu all over again … He felt if he were acquitted in the euthanasia case, no one would ever challenge anything he did again … It was a major miscalculation and a terrible mistake …
>
> What he never realised, or admitted to, was that most people aren't very rational, society isn't very rational. He had moved society more than he had any right to expect and further than anyone would have thought. By 1999 what he did was accepted in Michigan and would have been accepted

elsewhere had he not pushed the envelope. He could even have admitted that he had done euthanasia on occasion and gradually that would also have been accepted. It is ironic that someone so entrenched in biology, missed the point that change is evolutionary as well as revolutionary.

Mistake number three was sending the tape of the euthanasia to the most popular newscast in America, *60 Minutes.* The tape he mailed to Mike Wallace for Sunday night airing on CBS revealed to all viewers Dr Death unequivocally inserting a needle into Thomas Youk's arm. In one fell swoop Jack raised the ante from assisted suicide to euthanasia, shocked the nation with his apparent detachment, gave the state concrete evidence to arrest and arraign him, have a jury convict him and ultimately have Judge Cooper sentence him to imprisonment in a state penitentiary.

Mike Wallace, CBS Commentator, wrote:

> I was surprised, candidly, about the conviction. I believed him to be, believed [sic], and still do, to be a compassionate man. He was willing, really, to put his own freedom at issue. Which speaks to certain bravery. He's a brave man, an educated man, a zealot.
>
> He's a fascinating man. I have met a lot of interesting individuals down the years, not all of whom, not all of whom [sic], have demonstrated the courage that he did.

Nonetheless, it wasn't one of Jack's finest hours. 'In retrospect one has to ask how Jack could have been so stupid as to push the envelope as he later did,' says attorney Michael Schwartz:

We already know the why; the how perhaps should be naïvety rather than stupidity, with a little ego thrown in.

He got it into his head that the only way for him to get true endorsement, to have the Supreme Court of the land sanction assisted suicide was to sacrifice his freedom and go to jail. There would be a populace popular groundswell, he would be vindicated and humanitarianism towards the sick and suffering would reign throughout the land. Gandhi went to jail. Martin Luther King Jr. went to jail. Galileo went to jail. Kevorkian would go to jail. What he forgot, or wished to forget, was that Gandhi and King had huge followings, organisations on the outside to make things happen, and it took the Catholic Church 350 years to forgive and condone Galileo. The groundswell never materialised and most people don't even know he's in jail, and perhaps don't care.

His further miscalculation was in both the sentence and in the venue of his incarceration. He thought he would be martyred for a year or two and incarcerated in a federal penitentiary. Wrong on both counts.

Jack's fourth mistake was his decision to represent himself at his next trial. He thought it was going to be his penultimate trial, as the Supreme Court would be his final judgment and justice would follow and reign supreme. The Supreme Court would legalise assisted suicide and inspire worldwide-legalised euthanasia.

Jack raged to whoever would listen that he was going to represent himself at the next *Michigan* v *Kevorkian* confrontation. His friends argued and pleaded to no avail. Jack felt he knew better. He thought he was smarter than Fieger, knew the law and knew

medicine. He could easily convince any panel that he was innocent faster and more succinctly than Attorney Geoffrey Fieger.
He accused his friends of deserting him, demanding they give
their support rather than argue. When Harry Wylie told Jack he
preferred not to spend the rest of his life visiting him in prison,
Jack rejoined that Harry was presumptuous in thinking he would
allow him visitation.

When he was summarily arrested for the murder of Thomas
Youk, Jack began to have second thoughts about sitting at the
bench alone for his defence. He needed the assistance of attorneys. He chose David J Gorosh and Lisa Dwyer and made his fifth
mistake.

David was very intelligent, but he had only been out of law
school a few years and this would be his first high profile case. He
was also the only attorney that would allow Jack defend himself,
offering himself up for counsel and advice if Jack got in trouble.
As Fieger later said, 'It was like having an amateur weekend ball
player perform in an All Star game.' Jack also hired Lisa Dwyer,
another young attorney, for counsel and advice, however she
played a relatively small role in his defence.

Many others in the legal field pleaded with Jack to let them
defend him properly, but Jack was certain he could, without too
much assistance, reach the jury and instil in them the power to
change the law, circumvent the bureaucracy, get past the elected
officials and make a difference in the way terminal patients were
to be treated.

At the start of the Youk trial, at a hearing held before the start
of jury selection, Judge Jessica Cooper asked Kevorkian, 'Do you
realise the risk involved, that you could spend the rest of your
life in prison?'

'There's not much of it left, your honour,' Kevorkian said. 'I intended to represent myself all along.'

Cooper then asked Kevorkian if he had ever seen the inside of a prison, if he understood the limitations of the questions he could ask witnesses and if he understood that he had to follow the rules of the court. Kevorkian said that he did, and that he intended to 'say nothing but the truth' during the trial. The judge then reluctantly granted his request.

The Tom Youk court case lasted only one-and-a-half days. In the lead-up to the case, Kevorkian became increasingly worried about his resolve. Fieger tried to advise him to get proper legal counsel, but Kevorkian was adamant. He was, after all, hoping to lose, but as the day neared he feared what would happen.

The case was a fiasco. Kevorkian made numerous factual errors regarding criminal law during his opening statement, and the judge had to stop him and ask the jury to leave the room.

In his opening statement, Kevorkian argued that he did not intend to kill Thomas Youk, but felt compelled by his duty as a physician to do so. He compared himself to an executioner, who has a job to do – a job that was legal and sanctioned by society. He also said that his purpose in doing what he did was to make his case for euthanasia in a court of law, stating that he wanted to 'get into this sanctum sanctorium where it is difficult to lie and get away with it'.

The legal problem with this was that Jack proposed to define malice as 'a vicious act that required a vicious will'. Prosecutor John Skrzynski objected, saying that Kevorkian was making a legal argument rather than just laying out the facts – something attorneys are not allowed to do in an opening statement. The judge strongly advised Kevorkian that he should confer with his lawyers before returning to his opening statement. He refused.

To prevent Kevorkian from presenting evidence about Youk's condition – and perhaps using the trial as a forum of debate over euthanasia – prosecutors had dropped the assisted suicide charge. Two days before, Judge Cooper had admitted testimony about pain and suffering, ruling that it was relevant to assisted suicide. When that charge was dropped, the testimony was no longer admissible. The jury would have to choose murder or acquittal.

Kevorkian's defence was shackled by the manoeuvre. Since the pain and suffering of Tom Youk was only relevant to assisted suicide and not to murder, Kevorkian was forced to rest his case without calling any witnesses. The prosecution, however, had the videotape and *60 Minutes* interview.

'This is a terrible disease, but those things are not the issue,' the prosecutor argued. 'The law does not recognise mercy killing as a reason to kill somebody.'

During closing arguments, Kevorkian told jurors that only he knew his true intent when he helped Youk die, that they could not infer his motives from the tapes. He claimed he was only doing his duty as a dedicated physician and following Youk's wishes to end his suffering.

'Thomas Youk didn't want to die … no one does,' Kevorkian said. 'But there are times when you must because of certain circumstances. The issue here is whether Tom wanted what was done and whether I committed murder in the process of my helping him. That's what you must decide.'

The facts presented reasonable doubt over whether he intended to kill Youk – that instead he was providing a medical service to Youk.

But in his closing arguments, the prosecutor said that the videotape – and the interview with CBS' *60 Minutes* – showed that

Kevorkian killed Youk to make a political statement on euthanasia. Playing parts of the tape for the jurors, he said that Kevorkian made the tape knowing he wanted it presented in a court of law and admitted it to *60 Minutes'* Mike Wallace.

> He has an agenda, to bring this issue before a court. He tells
> Mike Wallace, 'They must charge me. Either they go or I go ...
> if they go that means they'll never convict me in a court of law.'
> He thinks that prosecutors will charge him with manslaughter,
> not necessarily murder. That shows that he knew he had killed
> a man.

He emphasised that Kevorkian's trial was not about Youk's illness, euthanasia or the debate over assisted suicide but about the reputed 'Dr Death's' right to kill. He pointed out to jurors that Kevorkian barely knew Youk 24 hours before he killed him. While playing the videotape of Youk's death, he said that Kevorkian did not even shut the deceased Youk's mouth before removing the needles hooking him to the medical devices. The implication was that Kevorkian was only concerned about killing Youk to advance his political agenda, not about the 52-year-old's well-being.

When the jury returned with its verdict, Kevorkian was found guilty of murder, contrary to the Prosecuting Attorney's recommendation, and sentenced to 10 to 25 years in prison.

The following is part of the statement made by Judge Jessica Cooper before sentencing Dr Jack Kevorkian to prison:

> This is a court of law and you said you invited yourself here
> to take a final stand. But this trial was not an opportunity for
> a referendum. The law prohibiting euthanasia was specifically

reviewed and clarified by the Michigan Supreme Court several years ago in a decision involving your very own cases, sir.

So the charge here should come as no surprise to you. You invited yourself to the wrong forum.

Well, we are a nation of laws, and we are a nation that tolerates differences of opinion because we have a civilised and a nonviolent way of resolving our conflicts that weighs the law and adheres to the law.

We have the means and the methods to protest the laws with which we disagree. You can criticise the law, you can write or lecture about the law, you can speak to the media or petition the voters.

But you must always stay within the limits provided by the law. You may not break the law. You may not take the law into your own hands …

No one is unmindful of the controversy and emotion that exists over end-of-life issues and pain control. And I assume that the debate will continue in a calm and reasoned forum long after this trial and your activities have faded from public memory.

But this trial is not about that controversy. The trial was about you, sir. It was about you and the legal system. And you have ignored and challenged the Legislature and the Supreme Court. And moreover, you've defied your own profession, the medical profession.

You stood before this jury and you spoke of your duty as a physician. You repeatedly speak of treating patients to relieve their pain and suffering. You don't have a licence to practice medicine. The state of Michigan told you eight years ago you may not practice medicine. You may not treat patients. You may not possess – let alone inject – drugs into another human being ...

Now, another consideration and perhaps even a stronger factor in sentencing is deterrence. This trial was not about the political or moral correctness of euthanasia. It was all about you, sir. It was about lawlessness. It was about disrespect for a society that exists and flourishes because of the strength of the legal system.

No one, sir, is above the law. No one ... You were on bond to another judge when you committed this offence, you were not licensed to practice medicine when you committed this offence and you hadn't been licensed for eight years. And you had the audacity to go on national television, show the world what you did and dare the legal system to stop you. Well, sir, consider yourself stopped.

According to Mayer Morganroth, Jack's present lawyer of account, the trial was full of errors and omissions:

> The travesty of the trial is that the system really failed him. This happens far too often in high profile situations such as Jack's.

According to Morganroth, Jack's lawyer could have attacked cause of death. When the aired tape is reviewed, Jack says, 'Now I'm going to initiate the medicine' and presses the plunger of the syringe. Jack then says, 'He gasps, and he's out.' About two minutes later he continues, 'Now the particular fluids are reaching him.' According to Morganroth:

There is no evidence he wasn't dead with the gasp and when the syringe was plunged. In pretrial discussions, the judge said it was a viable defence, but when it came to trial there was no expert testifying and no evidence whatsoever showing Thomas Youk was probably dead when the sera was administered. The death certificate even registered that the cause of death was ALS.

The most significant mistake, says Morganroth, was that Jack's lawyer:

> ... contrary to the advisement from Jack and greater legal minds, made the motion to dismiss the assisted suicide charge. Apparently his thought was that they would never convict Jack of murder. The motion was filed and they had a hearing in front of the judge. She was clearly concerned and asked if he was sure that was what he wanted to do ... She cautioned him that if he went ahead he couldn't put in any evidence for pain, suffering and the mental state of the deceased. This could only come in under assisted suicide. He still said yes so she denied his motion. The prosecution, hearing that, two weeks later dismissed the charge of assisted suicide.

This meant that Kevorkian's only defence was that the service he rendered should be legal. But as she had stated, the judge did not allow any family members to testify as to Youk's wishes. Jack's state of mind *for intent* was never shown because of his inability to have witnesses to attest to these truths. The prosecution was able to argue without any witnesses and solely based on the tape, that Jack was an insensitive murderer.

The prosecutor also argued that Kevorkian had seen only limited medical data before the fact. Jack's thorough investigative
process, where he saw all the medical material and interviewed
the patient and his family, was never revealed.

The final error Morganroth notes was that the prosecutor stated,
'He can't testify now. He could have ...' The judge stopped him
before he could finish the statement. The prosecutor continued to
say that Kevorkian 'could testify' at least 12 more times. Prosecutors may not criticise defendants' opting not to testify in front of
jurors because that is their constitutional right under the Fifth
Amendment – the comment was sufficient grounds for a mistrial.
Kevorkian's lawyer didn't object to this until after the jury had
begun deliberating, and the judge ruled it was too late.

Judge Cooper imposed her sentence despite the heartfelt letter she
received from Thomas Youk's widow. Melody Youk wrote, in part:

> Dear Judge Cooper,
>
> I am the wife of Thomas William Youk, client of Dr Kevor-
> kian. As you know, I had looked forward to addressing the
> Court during proceedings ... However, I believe certain infor-
> mation may in fact be relevant to your considerations regarding
> sentencing, and thank you for taking the time to review the
> enclosed.
>
> I wish first to clarify that it was at my husband's request that
> Dr Kevorkian was contacted. Dr Kevorkian responded to that
> request, he did not initiate or solicit the contact.
>
> I believe that understanding how Tom lived his life is integral
> to understanding how it is that he came to choose to contact
> Dr Kevorkian.

Born in 1946, Tom worked throughout his life, starting with a paper route at age ten. He had worked as a chef's assistant, a hospital orderly and was to be trained as an auto mechanic when he was served a draft notice in 1966. He joined the Air Force, where he received excellent marks in training, certificates for outstanding achievement and had one of the highest security clearances. He was honorably discharged as Sergeant from the reserves in 1968. He went to college, earned a degree and made his living as an accountant until the last few years of his life. Some of the things that most troubled him were people who were dishonest, did not pull their share, or did not follow the rules, to the detriment of others.

I offer this information not only to establish that he was a responsible law abiding citizen of no small distinction but further, to show that he approached his illness as he had approached everything else in his life, with curiosity, determination and a problem solving response ...

He had come to the situation where; in addition to reaching the point of only being able to control his thumb and first two forefingers on his right hand, he was losing his ability to speak. In spite of receiving specific medications for these problems, he was having trouble swallowing and was choking. He had a food tube inserted directly into his stomach in late August, however was not metabolizing the food, as his bodily functions were apparently shutting down. He discovered that his lung capacity had dropped to 25% of his normal, but had determined for himself that he did not wish to be on a ventilator, nor completely dependant on others, in a totally paralyzed body.

I was devastated to realise that in spite of all our efforts, we had come near the end. I was crushed by his decision, but came to realise it was selfish for me to not to support him in his decision. He was not depressed, nor was he a victim. He requested Dr Kevorkian's help, was grateful for it and therefore could never have been the complainant, as suggested by the prosecution, in any action against Dr Kevorkian ...

Dr Kevorkian questioned Tom many times as to his resolve and determined, that in fact Tom was certain of his desire to have the doctor help him to relieve his suffering. I do not agree with the suggestion by the prosecutor, as surmised from the tape, that the doctor seemed cold, clinical or detached.

Of course, I wish that I had been able to speak at the trial, feeling that would have given the jury an opportunity to receive a more balanced view of the facts, but understood the prosecution's concern for a jury nullification based on Tom's situation of being near death.

However, not being able to speak did not allow us an opportunity to address the question of why Tom would have chosen the direct injection over assisted. Tom's sum of body control had been reduced to the limited movement of his thumb and forefinger of his right hand and his mind and appreciation of all things mechanical, found the more fail-safe direct injection left less to chance for an incomplete event.

On another point to my understanding, the jury was left with little choice. At a conference held on February 22, 1999 at the University of Michigan Law School titled The Press, the Law and Public Policy, Coroner Dragovic spoke to describe that there are only three categories as relates to death cause: natural, by your own hand and homicide. Clearly, there needs to be another category, as in Tom's situation.

This act ... was my husband's acknowledged choice and harmed no one other than himself. My husband was grateful for the doctor's assistance to relieve his suffering and hasten his passing. Tom was not a victim, and to his mind this was not a crime, and most certainly not murder.

I appeal to you on behalf of my husband, myself, and our families, to consider all of the foregoing aspects of the background provided herein and ask that you show compassion as well to Dr Kevorkian in your sentencing. He is a man who is honored by many for having the courage to stand up for them without regard for his personal jeopardy ...

And it may be that the event which has brought us together in this court, may not be illegal in our foreseeable future.

Perhaps allowing a clemency to a man in our present.

Melody Haskin Youk

Jack had made a deal with the prosecutor that he would be sent to a federal penitentiary, one of the 'country clubs' of the prison system where he could keep his keyboard, computer and flute, and have access to a capacious library. He had naïvely believed that once convicted he would get a minimal sentence of a couple of years, and that it would take only a few months for his case to reach the Supreme Court and make legal history by being acquitted once and for all of assisted suicide and euthanasia.

Instead, he received 10 to 25 years in state prisons. His expectations of prison life and the appeal courts turned out to be vastly awry.

Chapter 13

Prisoner # 284797

Jack had gone full circle from the time decades ago when he went to Columbus, Ohio in his '56 Ford to interview condemned prisoners and was repelled and shocked by man's inhumanity to man. He was now part of this appalling system.

On April 13th, 1999, immediately following his sentence, Jack was transported by paddy wagon to Jackson Prison, about 100 miles from the courthouse. It was a cold, rainy day. Jack was shackled wrist and ankle and wore his little hat and lightweight blue windbreaker. He said it was the most miserable moment he ever experienced in his 70 years of life.

As he shuffled along a walkway, two storeys above the main floor where the inmates were pacing and mingling, one of the inmates recognised him and shouted a cry of recognition and encouragement. This seemed to be picked up by the entire population, and they all cheered him on, 'Hey, Jack, we're with you, Jack. Go, Jack, go! Go, Jack, go!', following with a vigorous ovation. They gave him encouragement and the determination to go on.

Two days later, Jack was transferred to Oaks Correctional Facility in Manistee, Michigan, a maximum-security prison. More than half of America's prison population resides in maximum-security prisons. Violence is omnipresent, exacerbated by gang activity, overcrowding and what former US Supreme Court Justice, Warren Burger once called 'the boredom and frustration of empty hours and pointless existence'.

It took several weeks of paper processing before he was allowed to have visitors. Harry and Arlene Wylie took their first trip in May that year; Neal and his second wife also visited Jack for their first time in May, on their way home from their honeymoon.

Manistee is about 50 miles north of the centre of Michigan, on Lake Michigan. It is a beautiful, grass roots American town frequented by boaters, vacationers and tourists, all primarily from the Chicago area of Illinois, 150 miles across the lake. Oaks Correctional Facility is a Level IV security facility (there are six levels of security in Michigan, Ionia Maximum Correctional Facility, for the criminally insane, being the only Level VI). Perimeter security at the prison comprises of double fences, electronic detection systems including monitor cameras, razor-ribbon wire, gun towers and a 24-hour patrol vehicle with armed personnel.

Visitors were required to fill out forms and were given a locker key, for which the state charged 25 cents, for their personal effects. They were then searched, stamped and paraded along many narrow corridors with steel-barred doors banging in front and behind.

They visited Jack through a floor-to-ceiling glass barrier, speaking into a telephone. There was only one phone, so that if more than one person wanted to speak to him, they had to hold the phone between them. When Jack became vociferous regarding the government, his trial or any number of other subjects that made him angry, he could be heard through the glass, no telephone necessary.

Jack wore a blue uniform with orange epaulettes, which he said represented his rank: as low as you could get. He was kept in his cell 23 hours a day, excluding three 20-minute meal breaks. His cell was at the very end, second tier. He was allowed a shower every day, as part of his one hour 'break'. He was by far the oldest inmate at Oaks – a few inmates were in their mid-forties, but the majority were in their twenties. There were, at the time, about 960 inmates and, according to Jack, the population was predominantly black.

Jack was pleased to be allowed bread, jelly and peanut butter in his cell, which he really liked. All printed material had to come out of the library, be supplied by the guards or ordered directly from the publishers. Jack reported that the guards treated him well, and brought him lots of magazines and newspapers.

During this time he received a considerable amount of mail from well-wishers, which often included a $10 or $20 cheque; he even received £1,000 from a supporter in England. As the state seized his assets under a law that allows the government to charge inmates for the cost of their imprisonment, he planned to use these donations for his appeals. Shortly after he was convicted, the state had gone after his nest egg. Under a settlement reached between then attorney general Jennifer Granhold and Kevorkian's attorney Mayer Morganroth in August 1999, the state was entitled to 90 per cent of his $31,155.54 in personal savings, plus 90 per cent of his $405 monthly pension from St John Health System. The state wanted to take his corporate account as well. This was Penumbra Inc, the non-profit corporation he had established years earlier for research and later for his defence.

Because it was non-profit, donations Jack received could be deposited tax-free into this account. It contained $77,176.82 that Kevorkian managed as a defence fund. Morganroth argued that would deny him sufficient funds to mount an appeal, so he was allowed to keep that money.

Jack felt unfairly treated, in general, and disappointed by Judge Cooper. He also expressed regret about his quarrel with Geoffrey Fieger, but believed that Geoffrey couldn't have altered events with the hand that he was dealt. But for the most part his morale was high. It might have been that his ascetic lifestyle contributed to his state of relative well-being. He said that it wasn't great to be incarcerated, but he could live with it.

At first Harry Wylie was forever trying to get Jack to write letters, more as a form of recreation for him than for the actual correspondence, but Jack resisted, saying that he detested writing letters. Those he did write show his upbeat spirits:

> Dear Harry & Arlene,
>   Thank you both for taking the time and trouble (with that <u>long</u> drive) to cheer me up with that very welcome visit.
>   Best wishes,
>   Jack
>   P.S.: Now you can't say that I never write to you!

Harry tried another tack and in June 1999 wrote to Jack with a question and answer format, allowing dotted spaces for response. Jack's response:

> H: Realising that you don't like to write: How are you feeling?
> J: 'Probably the only place where a man can feel really secure

is in a maximum security prison, except for the imminent threat of release.' (Germaine Greer, Australian feminist writer, born 1939)

H: Is there any indication when you will be transferred?

J: 'One can always have one's boots on and be ready to leave.' (Michel de Montaigne, 1533–92.) I am ready.

H: Would you like for us to call Flora?

J: 'The pleasure we derive from doing favors is partly in the feeling it gives us that we are not altogether Worthless.' (Eric Hoffer, Amer. Philosopher, 1902–83) Yes, thanks.

H: If yes, what would you like for us to tell her?

J: 'Worry is interest paid on trouble before it falls due.' (W.R. Inge, Dean of St. Paul's, London, 1850–1954)

'You cannot fight against the future. Time is on our side.' (W.E. Gladstone, 1809–98)

H: Is there anyone else you would like us to contact?

J: 'He that has once done you a kindness will be more ready to do another than he whom you yourself have obliged.' (Benjamin Franklin, 1706–90) No, thanks.

H: If yes, what would you like us to tell them?

J: I said, 'No, thanks.'

H: If yes, what would you like us to ask them?

J: Didn't you hear me?!

H: Could you copy down a few of your most favorite adages, and who said them?

J: 'It's the friends you can call up at 4 a.m. that matter.' (Marlene Dietrich)

'Some folks are wise, and some otherwise.' (Tobias Smollett, Scot novelist, surgeon, 1721–1771)

'Macho doesn't mean mucho.' (Zsa Zsa Gabor)

'When you're angry, count to four; when you're very angry, swear.' (Mark Twain)

H: Could you copy down a few of your Limericks?

J: Whenever I write you at home

From here, or wherever I roam,

You must understand

What you now have in hand

Is the closest you'll get to a tome!

Propitious wishes,

Jack

The Armenian community in Michigan never forgot Jack. A group of his second generation childhood friends meet weekly to this day. Although Jack held them at arm's length, as he did many people, those who were enthusiastic about his work treated him like family. A letter from Jack, again in June 1999, shows him welcoming their support:

What a nice and very welcome surprise to receive your card with all the signatures, comments, and best wishes from the good old South Side group! What fond memories it evoked, – sort of melancholy, in a way, how fast time has slipped by. The card definitely cheered me up.

I'm coping fairly well. It's much like the army, only less freedom. We get one hour 'yard' (outside to walk & exercise), 3 twenty meal breaks, & a 10 minute shower. Otherwise, always in the cell – a bare 10' x 12' room, 1 window, steel door with small window, concrete bed and shelf (for writing), a thin mattress, 2 sheets, 2 blankets. No chair, no desk. A small metal sink – toilet unit. One can get used to it. Food fair, usually enough of it. Inmates have been pretty respectful. No trouble if one follows the rules. The worst part is boredom. I'll probably be transferred soon to minimum-security facility where I can be much busier & constructively occupied. Here I can receive nothing but letters, cards or a few news clippings – no stamps, stationery, books, food, or gifts.

Please convey my gratitude & best wishes to the whole gang. I look forward to joining you all at those Monday sessions, and hopefully soon. Thank you again!

Murad

(υηιρωυ)

Despite the positivity, Jack was looking wan and thin. In August 1999, his blood pressure was recorded at 220 over 170. He had a fluttering in his chest and was feeling lightheaded; he demanded a check-up from the nurse and then the doctor, which due to red tape involved long delays. When he then requested that he be examined his own physician, Stan Levy, he was told to put him on his visitation list. After Jack arranged this, Stan was able to prescribe a change of medication and get his pressure down to 170 over 80. Jack has a tremendous fear of stroke. His brother-in-law Hermann had had one the previous year. Flora and Hermann had moved back to Michigan and bought a house not far from Jack's. Flora enjoyed being near her brother, but after Hermann's stroke, the medical costs drove the couple back to Germany – because of this, because of the free medication and treatment Jack received in prison, he felt that his incarceration was saving his life.

At the end of August, Jack was transferred to Kinross Correctional Facility in the Upper Peninsula of Michigan, a Level II security prison further from his home and friends. Prison officials asked him if he thought he would be able to go into the general population, and he answered positively. Almost immediately he regretted his decision, when he realised he would have to share a cell with two others. His roommates were murderers, sentenced to life without parole. It seemed that they were put in the same cell because they were all close in age, the other two prisoners being 62 and 57. Jack had to be in his cell only four times a day, for the rest of the time he could move about the facilities at will, both inside and out in the yard. Visitors were able to actually sit in the same room as Jack, although this meant Jack's pat down was more rigorous. Jack was feeling hopeful when first transferred, as his lawyers had just applied for his bond and parole. He expected a response in two to three weeks and was optimistic.

In fact Jack wasn't to stay there very long, but it was because of another transfer, this time to Charles Egeler Correctional Facility in Jackson, Michigan, a Level I security facility, primarily for infirm prisoners. In August 2000, after an appeal by attorney Michael Morganroth, Jack was moved again, this time to a Level II prison at Lapeer, Michigan: the Thumb Correctional Facility, which was closer to where most of his friends lived and made it easier for them to visit. Though this was a higher-level security prison, the rules there were slightly different. Jack still had to room with another inmate, but was allowed more time out of his cell.

In December 2000, the Michigan Supreme Court, without comment or review, denied Jack's bond, but allowed him to appeal to the United States Federal System – which meant he could take his case to the Supreme Court, his original goal. The previous

September, Jack had written to the individual Federal Supreme Court Justices raising the issue between court sanctioned executions and euthanasia. The letter read, in part:

> The issue of medical euthanasia, or physician aid in dying, is now of prime importance in the United States and several other countries. Clarification of its relation to rights and laws is urgently needed. Is the procedure to be governed by a capricious farrago of variegated state laws, or is it to be accorded the exalted status of a uniform, all-pervasive constitutional sanction? ...
>
> Medical art and science are entirely secular and serve a dual purpose: to lengthen life and to preserve or enhance its quality. Theoretically both aims are equally important, but arbitrary (and mainly sectarian) bias fostered an obsession to prolong life, no matter how inimical to its quality. The benefits of medicine permit its practitioners to perform acts that ordinarily are crimes. Thus we condone and even laud surgical mutilation ... as well as the occasionally nearly lethal poisoning of chemotherapy. The resultant quality of life is always subordinate to the chief aim of prolonging it. Why shouldn't the ranking sometimes be reversed? Why should we not just as readily condone and laud the chief aim of expunging – humanely, quickly, and with certainty – an intolerably low quality of individual life through a medical act ordinarily deemed to be homicide?
>
> Medical euthanasia was honorable and widely practiced in ancient Hippocratic Greece but later criminalized by the Church. The Renaissance philosopher-scientist Francis Bacon advocated that 'the medical profession should be permitted to ease and quicken death where the end would be otherwise only

delayed for a few days and at the cost of great pain.' In seventeenth-century England Sir Edward Coke, a distinguished lawyer and judge, dismissed charges against a physician who openly performed euthanasia. It was Coke's dictum that 'how long soever it hath continued, if it be against reason, it is of no force in law.' Accordingly, the long-continued criminalization of euthanasia is of no force because it is flagrantly against reason.

Almost two centuries later Thomas Jefferson advocated the use of a drug to end the terminal suffering from 'the inveterate cancer.' In 1910 Mark Twain asked his physician to end his suffering from heart disease. Dr Sigmund Freud's terminal agony, and also in 1936 that of England's King George V, ended with injections by their personal physicians, both vociferous advocates of the practice. The late distinguished American physician and author Dr Walter Alvarez several decades ago published his strong endorsement of medical euthanasia. Today more than half of all American physicians and an overwhelming majority of the public favor decriminalization of the practice, and a significant number of physicians admit to performing it furtively …

For the sake of unnecessarily suffering humanity I respectfully implore your High Court to exercise its prerogative under the supreme authority of the Ninth Amendment by validating as constitutionally protected the choice of suffering patients to request medical euthanasia and the choice of physicians to assess all aspects of that request and to honor it according to stringent guidelines. This right is as fundamental as that of life or liberty, and is certainly worthy of being the first right officially empowered through the Ninth Amendment. Concurrently it is essential that a commission of highly respected physicians be impaneled to establish the guidelines.

As a secular profession medicine is relevant to the full spectrum of human existence from conception *through* death. Any arbitrary legal constriction of that relevance is irrational, cruel, and barbaric. As guardians of human rights, you and your colleagues have the authority, opportunity, and obligation to rid society of this lingering medieval malady by using the Ninth Amendment to guarantee this most precious and humane *right of choice* for all Americans.

Sincerely and respectfully,

Jack Kevorkian, MD

Egeler Correctional Facility

Jackson, Michigan

This letter was subsequently published in the July 15th, 2001 issue of the *New York Review of Books,* when Mike Wallace of *60 Minutes* sent it to the editors in connection with the case of Timothy McVeigh, the man who set the bomb which killed 168 people at the Federal Building in Oklahoma City, Oklahoma on April 19th, 1995. Wallace noted that McVeigh had asked that he be put to death by lethal injection – a method that would use the same three chemicals Dr Kevorkian used in the death of Thomas Youk. He also noted that McVeigh had killed 168 innocent people, while Dr Kevorkian had assisted one person who – along with his wife and brother – had pleaded with Jack to help him end his suffering. Wallace went on to write:

Why do I raise all this again now? Because of the apparent irony: McVeigh and Youk, both of them wanting to die, and by the same means. But Thomas Youk's killer did what he did out of compassion, unlike McVeigh who killed out of bitterness. As

I've come to know more about Jack Kevorkian over the past two years, I've learned that the conventional wisdom about him was wrong. Fanatic? No. Zealot? Yes.

Meanwhile ... Kevorkian has not been able to talk to the press about any of this, for the Michigan Corrections Commissioner has turned down all requests from reporters who want to see him in prison. Timothy McVeigh has been allowed to make statements to reporters since his conviction. Jack Kevorkian has been silenced since his.

Wallace was referring to the fact that in the summer of 2000, ABC News waged a court battle against the Michigan Department of Corrections to allow Barbara Walters to interview Kevorkian for her television programme *20/20*. Corrections invoked a state prisons policy that took effect in March 1999, barring television crews except for stock footage and scenes of inmates taking part in prison activities. A county circuit judge found in favour of ABC on July 13th, saying that the prison policy infringed on First Amendment Rights. However, two weeks later the ruling was blocked by a state appellate court.

On September 11th, 2001, Michigan Appellate Court began hearing Dr Kevorkian's case. The defence – he allowed Mayer Morganroth to defend him this time – maintained that Kevorkian's trial was inconsistent with the constitution, and asked that the court either retry him on a bond, or set him free. They also claimed that Jack's defence attorney, David Gorosh, did not help him enough during his trial. Forty minutes into the proceedings the hearing was interrupted and it was announced that the World Trade Center had just been attacked and the court was ordered to evacuate the building. Two months later, even though the hearing had been cut short, the appellate court decided against retrying Dr Kevorkian. The court refused Jack's claim against David Gorosh, saying that Kevorkian had demanded to represent himself while ignoring the trial judge's repeated reminders of the consequences. 'Defendant chose – almost certainly unwisely but nevertheless knowingly, intelligently, voluntarily, and unequivocally – to represent himself,' the appeals wrote. 'He cannot now assign the blame for his conviction to someone who did not act as his trial counsel.'

Jack also argued in his appeal that the trial judge acted improperly by not allowing testimony from Youk's widow. But the appellate court wrote that the testimony was irrelevant, that it had nothing to do with the case.

Jack's trial lasted a day and a half; his appeal forty minutes.

When a further appeal to the Supreme Court of Michigan was denied, Mayer Morganroth petitioned the 6th District Court in Cincinnati to expedite his plea for justice, but they too refused to read or accept his case. It appeared that Jack would finally have his wish at last, a reading by the Supreme Court of the United States. He had two tenets he wanted the Supreme Court to review:

1. The fundamental right of the terminally ill and suffering to have the right to choose how and when they die.
2. To establish rigorous safeguards against the abuse of physician power by legalising assisted dying.

After all Jack's planning, albeit misplaced, the Supreme Court refused to grant him certiorari – ie they would not review the lower court's decision. They said they would not hear his case without reason even though in a previous case, *Glucksberg v Washington*, the four Justices said they would like to hear a particularised case of assisted suicide wherein a person was in irremediable pain, and terminal. The Thomas Youk case was just such a case.

Jack's dream of getting assisted suicide and euthanasia acquitted in the Supreme Court had failed, and all that was now left – unless his sentence was commuted by the governor – was for Jack to sit out his time until he was paroled.

Jack's health suffered a great deal throughout his incarceration. In October 2003, Jack had a cold, atrophic spots on the brain, a double hernia and complained of double vision (actually quadruple vision, as he sometimes saw four walkways and had difficulty walking because he didn't know which path to tread). He was lethargic and had on-and-off headaches.

Jack finally convinced the authorities to take him to the hospital in Jackson Penitentiary, where the main prison hospital for Michigan is located. It was a two-hour drive both ways and he was shackled with both leg irons and handcuffs. He fell getting out of the van and scraped his hands and arms. The trip back took five-and-a-half hours because the wagon had another pick-up at Oaks before the trip back to the Thumb. The trip involved four strip searches.

For his trouble, however, the doctor changed his blood pressure medication which improved most of his symptoms.

It took seven weeks before Jack was fitted with a truss for his hernia and two more years before the state afforded corrective surgery.

Jack summed up his plight in one of his Limericks:

Autonomy – what we all crave

As a birthright through life to the grave

Is but a vain quest

In this land that's oppressed

By tyrants hell-bent to enslave.

Although he may have thought differently, Jack was not forgotten by the outside world. In April 2004 the Michigan Armenian community circulated the following petition to be mailed, individually, by concerned citizens:

Date _____

Governor Jennifer Granholm

State Capital

PO Box 30013

Lansing, MI 48909

Honorable Governor Granholm,

As of April 13, 2004 Dr Jack Kevorkian completed five years of a 10–25 year prison sentence for mercifully ending the life of a fellow human being who begged Dr Kevorkian to end the excruciating pain and suffering caused by Lou Gerhig's [sic] disease.

In March 2004, Carol Carr, a resident of the State of Georgia was released from a Georgia prison after serving 21 months of a five year sentence for shooting to death her two adult sons who were suffering from Huntington's disease. It was a merciful act by a desperate loving mother.

Although both deeds were similar, Dr Kevorkian's punishment seems to be more cruel and unusual. Is it because the citizens of Michigan are less compassionate? Less understanding? Less forgiving? I don't think so, therefore I am joining the 'FREE DR. JACK' campaign in pleading to you for the immediate commutation of his sentence.

It's the humane thing to do. Please Governor, 'FREE DR. JACK'.

Compassionately Yours,

Signature

Printed Name _____

Street _____

City _____ State _____

Zip _____

Also, on April 11th, 2004, Carol Poenisch, an elementary school teacher and daughter of Merian Frederick, was quoted in the *Oakland Press*:

The sentence was too long, too severe; he's served his time.

He helped relieve her suffering. It was really difficult, wanting to save her and at the same time giving her what she wanted – that autonomy, that choice. In a way, it's how much I loved her; how I tried to be the best daughter I could be.

I try to send him books to read – he likes nonfiction, historical books, things with a little bit of controversy.

I think he's a man with a lot of courage. I wouldn't agree with the way he does everything, but I trust Jack. Nobody else would do what he's done. Every cause needs a maverick like that.

The same *Oakland Press* article quotes Jack as saying:

There's no doubt I expect to die in prison. All the big powers ... they've silenced me ... So much for free speech and choice on this fundamental human right. The American people are sheep. They're comfortable, rich, working ... It's like the Romans, they're happy with bread and their spectator sports. The Super Bowl means more to them than any right.

Look at the forces against me – the government, the American Medical Association, pharmaceutical companies and religion. Is there anything more powerful than these four?

The journalist asked, 'What is the worst part about prison?'

Jack responded, 'It's the boredom that kills you. You read until you're tired of that. You do crossword puzzles until you're tired of that. This is torture. This is mental torture.'

When asked if he's doing OK, Kevorkian laughed. 'No,' he said. 'People ask me that all the time, and I always say, "No! No!"'

Appreciating moral support, but remaining fatalistic:

There is nothing anyone can do anyway. The public has no power. The government knows I'm not a criminal. The parole board knows I'm not a criminal. The judge ... knows I'm not a criminal.

I failed in securing my options for the choice for myself, but I succeeded in verifying the Dark Ages is still with us. When history looks back, it will prove what I'll die knowing.

Chapter 14

VISCUS

Imprisonment may have cost Jack Kevorkian his freedom, but it has never, and will never, stop his pursuit of ideas to help relieve people's suffering and ill health – no matter how radical these ideas may be. While in prison, Jack resumed his research on the topic of organ transplants. He focused on the statistics and circumstances surrounding the organ shortage that has plagued the United States in recent years. Although medical science has created numerous advances in the techniques employed in organ transplantation, Jack was dismayed by the systemic flaws that limit the availability and distribution of organs.

Organ transplant had been one of Jack's 'causes' since his early idea of using organs from condemned criminals. In 1998, he received permission from a 45-year-old patient named Joseph Tushkowski to harvest his kidneys for transplantation after his death. Protected by infusion of a patented solution and placed under refrigeration, they were usable for transplantation for up to 48 hours. Although the Michigan medical examiner LJ Dragovic stated that the kidney removal was carried out with a blatant disregard for the rules and regulations of organ procurement, saying,

'The kidneys were taken out after death. They were totally useless and not procured properly,' in fact, the kidneys were removed at the moment following the cessation of Joseph's heart. He had been dead only moments – and the transplantation of cadaver organs has been done for many years.

The organs were offered to any patient who could get their transplant surgeon to use them. Jack went on television pleading for a surgeon somewhere in the US to take the organ to save someone's life. Jack and Neal Nicol manned the phones throughout the night. There were many calls, but they were all from patients and patients' loved ones. Jack and Neal referred them to their transplant surgeons, who evidently rejected the idea.

No one received the kidneys, and they were consequently buried with the patient. Two patients may have died because of the indifference of the transplant society.

In his research, Jack found that approximately 17 patients die needlessly every day in the United States waiting for their 'miracle', an organ transplant. On any given day, nearly 82,000 anguished patients in the United States wait, often in vain, for an organ transplant that could save their lives, or at least improve their quality of life. More than 6,000 of these people die waiting, while thousands more suffer in great distress waiting for an organ to become available. Many people are not even eligible to be put on the waiting lists because, due to the organ shortage, they are considered too sick to receive an organ.

Unfortunately, it is estimated that only one of every ten families of 20,000 brain-dead, heart-beating patients consent to organ donation of loved ones. This shortfall represents a loss of organs from more than 18,000 contributors. There are potentially six life-saving organs per donor: two kidneys, one liver, one heart and two lungs, representing the distressing loss of a possible 108,000 organs per year.

As of 1984, it is illegal in the United States to give or make money from transplants. In that year the National Organ Transplant Act was passed whereby individuals are liable a $50,000 fine and five years in prison for the conviction of purchasing or selling organs. Not everyone agrees that paying for organs is a bad idea. Nicolas Kristof, a Pulitzer Prize-winning writer for the *New York Times*, wrote in November 2002 that the reason people die waiting for organs is not just failed kidneys or hearts, but:

> ... failed policy – specifically, the ban passed in 1984 by Congress on payment for organs. A debate erupted in the medical community this year on this issue, and by the time the policy is overturned – as it will be – it'll have killed more Americans than the Vietnam War ... One problem with the existing system is that the shortage means many live people donate spare kidneys to needy relatives. At least two live donors died in the past three years because of the surgery, and a third was left in a vegetative state. Moreover, paying for organs would be cost-effective, because dialysis costs much more than transplants.

In September of 1993, a seller from Sunrise, Florida, posted an ad on eBay that said, 'A fully functional kidney for sale. You can choose either kidney. Buyer pays all transplant and medical costs. Of course, only one is for sale, as I need the other one to live.' The bidding started at $25,000 and topped off at $5,750,000. When eBay officials got wind of the auctioning, they removed the item from their site. There were seven bidders, obviously so desperate to get the help they needed that they were willing to bid for a human organ from a total stranger.

But there are ways to obtain organs on the black market for those with the financial means. A burgeoning, lucrative market presently exists in underground organ commerce. Turkey and India are two of the largest purveyors of organs while Iraq, prior to the war, transplanted 600 kidneys annually. China, Russia and even the US are diligently involved in the swapping of human organs. Jack noted that this illegal process has many perils: the possibility of unsanitary harvesting and transplantation facilities, the questionable capabilities of the medical practitioners, offensive advantages taken by the rich upon the poor, unsavoury organ brokers, the cloak and dagger irregularity of the bartering process and the illegal practice in general. He concluded that if kidney sales were legalised, brokers and rogue physicians would be out of business, and money could flow to sellers and research.

Jack's research also recognised that between 1990 and 1999, despite numerous marketing efforts trying to persuade people to sign donor cards, the US organ waiting lists grew five times as fast as the number of organs donated. By the year 2010 it is estimated that the average wait for a kidney will exceed ten years.

According to Dr Richard Rohrer, the chief of transplant surgery at New England Medical Center in Boston, a person who receives a living-donor kidney has a reasonable hope of a lifetime of kidney function, whereas a person with a cadaveric kidney has a reasonable hope of a decade of kidney function.

Traditionally, organ donation has been viewed as an act of altruism. You should register to donate your organs because doing so can save a life; that should be the only reward you need. That may be so, but such thinking has failed to convince potential donors.

The present altruistic donation system, operated by the United Network of Organ Sharing (UNOS), does not work. According to their own statistics, 2,583 Americans died in 2000 waiting for a kidney. Worldwide, the number of annual deaths is estimated to be at least 50,000. This is for renal requirements only; needs for lungs, hearts, and livers (and potentially pancreases) would be exponential.

The May 2002 edition of *Red Herring*, a monthly publication covering the business of technology, stated that in 2001, just 23,000 organs were available for 74,000 on transplant waiting lists. The article also noted that:

> The law says if you want to die and are terminally ill, we won't let you, you have to live. But if you want to buy an organ that will allow you to live, we won't let you; you'll have to die. How incongruous the law is.
>
> Because organ scarcity is an economic problem, as well as a medical and moral one, market-based incentives offer the best means of alleviating the organ shortage. An organ market would attract the capital needed to accelerate the progress of research in this area. It would also help ensure that organ transplants are covered by health insurance providers and national health care systems, are regulated for abuse, and are cleansed of some of their ghoulishness.

According to Dr Michael Friedlaender, a nephrologist at Hadassah University Hospital in Jerusalem, the system is a free-for-all.

Instead of turning our backs on this, instead of leaving our patients exposed to unscrupulous treatment by uncontrolled free enterprise, we as physicians must see how this can be legalised and regulated. The current system of organ donation without remuneration is a failure.

Jack Kevorkian, as always, was ahead of his time. While in prison he has developed a system to eliminate the shortage of transplantable human organs by means of a free, non-profit, nationwide, ultimately global, on-line auction market. Finally receiving recognition from the medical establishment, in 2001, the entire 80-page issue of the *American Journal of Forensic Psychiatry* (Volume 22, Issue 2) was devoted to an article by Jack entitled, 'Solve the Organ Shortage: Let the Bidding Begin'. This treatise was written with little library assistance and no internet access. He did, however, open his own internet site www.viscus.org, with the assistance of Harry Wylie (viscus means vital organs). This site is still available for access.

In his paper, Jack argued that 'commercialisation of transplantable human organs is the only sure way to end the crisis of their supply. This is best accomplished by implementing a free, non-profit, nationwide, ultimately global on-line auction market.'

Jack advocates that an attempt to set prices through countless individual one-on-one negotiations would be unseemly, time-consuming, chaotic and essentially unworkable. The solution, he feels, lies in a free on-line auction similar to the efficient supply–demand process of computerised securities and commodity exchanges. The auction could be well organised and monitored and smoothly operational if it is free of 'governmental, political, academic, sectarian, or other bureaucratic control'.

Jack envisages the process to work this way:

Someone on a life support is medically determined brain-dead. The family donates the organs for transplantation and the organs go on auction on the internet as any other commodity might on eBay.

The first objection most people have to this plan is that only the rich would be able to afford transplantation. Jack has answers to this: two-thirds of the income derived from selling these organs would be placed in escrow, available to medical institutions that could bid on the next offering for the indigent. In this manner everyone would eventually have fair access to donated organs, the rich because they can afford it, and the poor because a fund had been established to accommodate them.

The remaining third would go to the donors' families or to charitable donations if they prefer. Approximately 1 per cent of the income would be used for administrative and operational costs.

Eventually, the economic capitalistic market would come into play. As more organs are donated, the organ shortage would ease and bid prices should drop to the further advantage of the indigent.

The issue included not only the article, but also commentary by a dozen surgeons, physicians and psychiatrists. While generally supporting the journal's decision to open the debate, several voiced serious objections to Kevorkian's proposal. Dr Martin S Zand and Dr Richard A Demme of the University of Rochester Medical Center, contended that the organ auction, 'raising millions of dollars for hospitals and donating families', would create a severe backlash, and that people would be afraid that hospitals might encourage physicians to declare their condition hopeless to 'procure their organs for lucrative financial remuneration' or that family members might be tempted to sell their organs instead of urging doctors to save their lives. The doctors stated:

> We strongly disagree with Dr Kevorkian's proposal to replace altruism with avarice as the motivation for organ donation. Our rebuttal consists of three major points: 1) The proposal will substantially decrease organ donation 2) it will lead to greater inequity in organ distribution and 3) it is technically unworkable.

In another commentary, Dr Albert M Drukteinis, MD, JD stated:

> We as a society should not, and more importantly we as physicians should not, become the instrument of death for whatever altruistic reasons. This is a fundamental shift from valuing life, to valuing death, even if as in organ auctioning, it is under the guise of prolonging life for others. In both physician-assisted suicide and organ auctioning, death is not only valued, but welcome and promoted.

Dr Ronald Shlensky, MD, JD countermanded with:

> Dr Kevorkian has apparently recognised that the current approach to the distribution of organs for transplantation is disorganised and replete with bias ...
>
> As psychiatrists we recognize that some constructive ideas are less than palatable and as physicians we have had to struggle with the proper balance between providing service and

making money. Many of us had both in mind when we chose the medical profession, studies have shown. This is probably 'human nature' but we can get beyond such natural forces if we push. There are times when reality and the welfare of others can marry.

Jack believes that there are many ancillary advantages to his system. Private funding through auctioning would ease the financial burden of, and the risks of litigation for, insurance and healthcare organisations and would reduce or eliminate the demeaning need to solicit, or beg for, funds to aid the uninsured. A marked increase in transplantation would mean that more surgeons would work more often to hone their skills and techniques, improve their results and earn higher incomes. There would be no extra cost to taxpayers. Otherwise idle private money would filter through and stimulate the nation's economy.

Shortly after the website was established, Harry Wylie mailed letters to major transplant surgeons, medical hospitals, medical research facilities and the media advising them of the *American Journal of Forensic Psychiatry* issue and directing them to the website for their suggestions and comments.

There wasn't a single response. Once again, despite the debate sparked in the journal, an idea of Jack's that will help millions of people has yet to reach a satisfactory conclusion.

While in prison Jack again picked up the gauntlet against capital punishment and for using condemned prisoners' organs for transplants. In April 2004, he mailed an 'open letter' to the governors of states still dispensing the death penalty, the state's major newspapers, Barbara Walters and Mike Wallace, saying that although he was generally opposed to capital punishment, he was asking the judiciary and the legislators to consider a 'valuable modification' in the way the death penalty was enforced – that modification being organ transplantation with the 'fully informed consent and choice' of the condemned. Jack ended the letter by saying:

> If you and your legislature are sincerely and irrevocably dedicated to the continuation of this nihilistic penalty, you now have an unprecedented opportunity to facilitate this almost miraculous extraction of life from death. It is up to you to prove that the spirit or essence of the political entity you represent still has some degree of residual nobility – at least enough to mitigate the vengeful perversion that is brazen judicial homicide.
>
> I have no doubt that posterity's judgment as to whether or not any society now using the death penalty is truly compassionate and rational will entail the latter's decision either to implement this proposed option immediately, or to abolish capital punishment immediately – and forever.

On a light-hearted note, Jack has also spent his time in prison to publish another book, this time a mélange of diversions called *glim^merIQs: a Floriligium*, a collection of thoughts, conceptions, repudiations and accomplishments most dear to him. Published in January 2004, it is a compendium of 180 Limericks; terse verses (eg, neurology – nervous service; gluttony – cloy ploy; gynaecologist – tender gender mender; pregnancy – womb bloom); a dissertation on quantum physics titled 'Beyond any Kind of God'; reproductions of his paintings; a selection of his music compositions, geometric dissection of the human body to assist pathological and forensic research as well as future robotic surgery; and an assemblage of digressions.

The book concludes with:

> For some this book's ending may be
> Sad yearning, for others pure glee;
> So your boos or hurrahs
> Won't affect me, because
> It's my liberating soliloquy.

The key word in the Limerick is 'liberating'. Jack continually talks about his liberation – not from prison, but from this life. He never mentions the word 'suicide', only 'it' – as in 'when I do it' or 'I'm going to do it soon' or 'I'll have you visit with Flora just before I do it'. 'It' is in reality suicide by starvation.

Chapter 15

LEGACY

Jack Kevorkian is used to fighting losing battles. The one he's fighting now may be his last.

In December 2005, prison doctors told Jack that the hepatitis C he contracted while researching cadaver blood transfusions more than 40 years ago has reached extremely dangerous levels. He is also suffering from high blood pressure, cardiovascular disease, temporal arthritis, peripheral arthritis, adrenal insufficiency, chronic pulmonary obstruction disease and cataracts. The American prison system is notorious for inadequate medical care, and Jack's case is no exception. He is now suffering not only the indignities of prison life, but also the indignities of having a major illness without proper medical attention. This is indeed cruel and unusual punishment for a man who has always maintained that he would take his own life rather than suffer to the end.

Attorney Mayer Morganroth applied to Michigan governor Jennifer Granholm to show compassion and grant a pardon and/or commutation of sentence for Dr Kevorkian, who is eligible for parole in 2007.

Although a December 2005 MSNBC national poll showed that 88 per cent of the people who participated believed Kevorkian should be freed, the Michigan state parole board obviously felt otherwise. On 22nd December, the board voted 7–2 to recommend denying the application. The board's recommendation then went to Governor Granholm, who had previously stated that she wouldn't consider pardoning him.

Jack Kevorkian is a physician who believes that people faced with intolerable pain as a result of disease or aging have a right to decide how much they have to bear before they leave this earth.

He is an idealist, who went into medicine to help humanity and found himself charting the unmapped regions of death. His ideas have had great potential to benefit millions; however, they are also ideas that shake social taboos and require too much of an emotional leap for many people to accept.

More important than his failures, though, is the fact that his attempts to save many, many patients the fear, pain and degradation of terminal illness have changed how we view death and dying. Universities are now teaching young doctors how to handle terminal situations. He has furthered the use of living wills, do not resuscitate orders, pain management, hospice care, palliative care and end-of-life concerns. He personally helped over 130 people to end their suffering from terminal illness and unbearable pain; many more people throughout the world are now quietly being helped by their doctors to die.

The press covers each of Dr Kevorkian's legal appeals, while his name is thrown around as shorthand for the right-to-die movement in talk shows on radio and television. When the media reported the Supreme Court's decisions on Oregon's

assisted suicide law, they immediately referred to Dr Kevorkian in order to provide context for the debate. The same thing
happened when, in a case that gripped the United States in controversy, Michael Schiavo asked Florida courts to permit him
to remove the feeding tube that kept his brain-dead wife, Terri
Schiavo, alive. Schiavo suffered brain damage in 1990 when her
heart stopped briefly due to a chemical imbalance that might
have been caused by an eating disorder. She could breathe on
her own, but relied on a feeding tube to keep her alive. Despite
the fact that several doctors declared her to be in a persistent
vegetative state with no hope of recovery, her parents continued
to insist that she could improve with treatment.

In a rare media interview (allowed because it was a phone conversation as opposed to cameras being brought into the prison),
Jack spoke to ABC's *Good Morning America* about the Schiavo case.
He was dismayed by what he saw as the hypocrisy of the politicians involved who argued 'life is sacred and must be preserved
at all costs', but who simultaneously favoured the death penalty.
However, Kevorkian said that he believed some good could come
from the debate over end-of-life wishes.

'It has raised the issue,' he said, 'and many more people [will] be
willing to face it and discuss with families and society in general.'

That is the legacy that Jack Kevorkian leaves the world. He
forced individuals and the country as a whole – indeed most of
the Western world – to look at death and dying not as a forbidden
subject, but as a fact of human existence about which we should
have the right to make choices and decisions, difficult though
they may be.

The day after the Schiavo's death, Dr John D Canine, a psychologist at Wayne State University in Detroit who has studied

the way people think about death, told the *Washington Post* (April 1st, 2005) that '… we don't like to think about the inevitable, which is that we're all terminal', and that the 'Kevorkian case and [the Schiavo] case have both pointed us to a mirror. We've had to look and see that our lives are very limited and that death is inevitable for all of us …'

The Schiavo case revisited a number of important issues that Jack Kevorkian first brought to wide public attention, the most evident being the value of living wills. In just three months from the time of Schiavo's death, Aging with Dignity, a non-profit organisation in Florida devoted to supporting end-of-life wishes, received requests for more than 800,000 copies of its Five Wishes form, which combines living wills with the appointment of a medical proxy (an individual with the power to make life-or-death decisions for another person). This was 60 times the normal number of requests.

One of the reasons the Schiavo case was so contentious was that Terri Schiavo did not have a living will. Michael Schiavo stated that his wife had told him she would not want to be kept alive in a vegetative state, but there was nothing in writing, and her parents contended that she never would have said such a thing. This kind of ambiguity is exactly what Jack sought to avoid by helping only those patients who were mentally alert and competent, and by videotaping their consultations so that there would be no question about their final wishes.

Schiavo's case brought home to millions of people what Jack had been fighting for so ferociously: the right of every individual to make his or her own decisions about end-of-life care. As medicine progresses, we lengthen human life without fully considering what is in a person's best interests. Jack Kevorkian consistently reminds us of this fact, and forces us to consider our own values in terms of quality of life and individual choice. This is what it was all about for Jack, and for Jack's patients and their families.

Another issue that was brought up by the fight to allow Terri Schiavo's feeding tube to be removed is one of the most divisive in the United States and around the world today. This is the struggle between two very different cultural perspectives: the conservative and mainly religious right that wants to control the body, and the progressive, liberal left that wants to cede control to the individual.

Between 1990 and 1998, when Jack was performing his assisted suicides, he faced opposition not only from the state, but from religious organisations as well, who would often picket in front of a courthouse where Jack was being tried. In 1998, during the second campaign to legalise assisted suicide in Michigan, the state's seven Catholic bishops issued a joint letter – for the first time in Michigan's history – that was mailed to all 550,000 Catholic households in the state, urging the faithful to vote 'no'.

In 2005, religious groups were a steady and visible presence outside the Florida hospice where Terri Schiavo lived. To Jack Kevorkian, politics and religion are two separate worlds that should not be used to determine each other's values. He conveyed his values on the subject in 1992, in his article in the *American Journal of Forensic Psychiatry* (Volume 13, Issue 1) where he stated that medicine was a secular profession '… like engineering and many others. It deals with health, disease, life and death in this empirical world. Religion has its centrepiece in the uninvestigable "world". The two worlds should co-exist without the intrusion of one on the other.'

In the United States, President Bush (himself a member of the Christian right) and his administration made it clear that they did not believe in the same sort of separation. Jeb Bush, the president's brother and the governor of the state of Florida, petitioned the court to have Schiavo taken into state custody so that he could have her feeding tube reinserted. An affidavit signed on behalf of the state by Dr William Cheshire, a board-certified neurologist at the Mayo Clinic in Minnesota, stated that his review of Schiavo's condition raised 'serious doubt' about her diagnosis. Dr Cheshire is also director of the Center for Bioethics and Human Dignity, a group founded in 1994 to recognise the contribution of 'biblical values' to the bioethical debate. The court refused the governor's petition.

The president himself got involved when he rushed back to the White House from his ranch in Crawford, Texas to sign a bill passed by the Republican Congress allowing Terri Schiavo's parents to ask a federal judge to order that Terri's feeding tube be reinserted. This order was also subsequently denied, and Schiavo passed away on March 31st, 2005.

The irony here, as well in the fight to uphold Oregon's Death with Dignity Act, is that conservative politicians have had to reverse one of their long-held philosophies – the belief in a limited role of government, with states' right privileged over centralised federal power. What Jack Kevorkian started as the crucial fight for an individual's control over his or her own body has grown into a battle over whether the federal government should have that right instead.

When Oregon was battling to pass the Death with Dignity Act, it aroused passionate opposition among political and religious conservatives. Bill Clinton, who was president at the time, and his administration, found that there was nothing in federal law that blocked the state from allowing assisted suicide. However, when George Bush was elected president, John Ashcroft, his attorney general, reinterpreted an already-existing law (the Controlled Substances Act) to make it a crime for physicians to prescribe lethal amounts of drugs.

When the justices at the US Supreme Court voted 6–3 to uphold the Oregon law, the religious right once again protested. Richard Land, president of the Southern Baptist Ethics and Religious Liberty Commission, told the *Baptist Press* (January 18th, 2006), 'It is sad that a majority of the current court prefers to see this issue in purely federal vs. state terms as opposed to the profound moral issue of involving the healing arts in death therapy ...' And David Stevens, executive director of the 17,000 member Christian Medical and Dental Association said in the same publication, 'Legalized assisted suicide gives doctors the right to help kill, and in our money-driven healthcare system, that's dangerous. The cheapest form of medical care is always a handful of lethal drugs.' This was countered by a statement from Barbara Lee Coombs, president of Compassion & Choices, an organisation that supports assisted suicide, who said the Court's decision '... reaffirms the liberty, dignity and privacy Americans cherish at the end of life. No government should threaten these rights nor usurp a state's power to meet the needs of its dying citizens.' But Richard Doerflinger, deputy director of pro-life activities for the US conference of Catholic Bishops, told the *Christian Century Magazine* in February 2006 that his organisation will ask Congress to clarify federal drug laws so assisted suicide can be forbidden.

Needless to say, the battle begun by Jack Kevorkian is far from over.

★

Of course, the United States is not the only forum for the debate on assisted suicide. In Australia, Dr Philip Nitschke, a vocal advocate and activist for assisted suicide and euthanasia, who is known there as Dr Death, is under intense government scrutiny. The law that makes it a crime to use a phone, fax, email, or Internet to access material that 'counsels or incites' suicide was passed specifically to stop Dr Nitschke's activities, after which Nitschke stated he planned to move his operation to New Zealand. The New Zealand government immediately began to investigate ways it might bar him entry. In the UK, over the past few years, Lord Joel Goodman Joffe has introduced into parliament a number of versions of the Assisted Dying for the Terminally Ill (ADTI) Bill. The version introduced in November 2005 allowed for assisting the dying, but not for voluntary euthanasia (which was included in earlier versions). This means that doctors, at the request of terminally ill patients, could prescribe life-ending medications but they would not be able to administer them.

The ADTI Bill is modelled on Oregon's Death with Dignity Act − which was modelled on Jack Kevorkian's principles of assisted suicide. The safeguards built into both the Oregon Act and the ADTI Bill are taken directly from the imperatives Kevorkian published in the *American Journal of Forensic Psychiatry* in 1992. Eligibility requirements for assisted suicide in the ADTI Bill are similar to those in Oregon: in order to receive medical help to die, a person would have to be terminally ill with six months or less to live; mentally competent; make persistent, well-informed, voluntary requests; and be suffering unbearably. Other safeguards include: patients have to make two oral and one written request for assistance in dying, to be verified by two witnesses other than family members; two independent doctors have to determine that the patient is well-informed and that the request is voluntary; patients must consult with a palliative care expert to explore alternatives; patients must wait at least 14 days before a request is granted; and patients can orally revoke the request at any point.

Lord Joffe was encouraged to introduce a new version of his bill, which had previously been defeated, when in July 2005 the British Medical Association (BMA) voted not to oppose the new bill. The BMA stated that the question of 'the criminal law in relation to assisted dying is primarily a matter for society and for Parliament'.

And in January of 2006, the *Daily Telegraph* reported that, according to a study conducted by Professor Clive Seale of Brunel University, nearly 3,000 patients in Britain were illegally helped to die by doctors in 2004. The survey showed that 936 of the 585,000 deaths in 2004 were described by doctors as voluntary euthanasia, while an additional 1,929 cases were described as 'ending life without an explicit request from the patient', which is also known as non-voluntary euthanasia.

As in America, pro-assisted suicide activists see its legalisation as a matter of personal choice. Tamora Langley of the Voluntary Euthanasia Society (now called Dignity in Dying) has stated that 'We must be allowed to make choices about what, for each of us, is a good death.' Public opinion in Britain seems to favour assisted suicide even more so than in the United States; a YouGov poll taken in November of 2004 showed that 80 per cent of Britons supported changing the law to make doctor-assisted suicide a legal option.

But the religious factions in the UK are just as vehemently opposed as they are in the US. In October 2005, nine leading figures from six major faith groups in the UK published a joint letter to both houses of parliament in a bid to lobby against legalising any form of assisted suicide or euthanasia. The letter warned parliament that the 'so-called "right-to-die" would inexorably become the duty to die and potentially economic pressures and convenience would come to dominate decision-making'. And in November of the same year, the Christian Medical Fellowship, which represents 5,000 doctors across the UK, released a statement opposing the Joffe Bill.

The question of assisted suicide was further fuelled in the UK in January 2006, when, as described in chapter 10, retired doctor Anne Turner travelled with her family to Switzerland, where assisted suicide is illegal only if the person assisting is acting out of self-interest.

The bishop of Oxford, the Right Reverend Richard Harries, told the BBC that he would want to convince a person who was considering assisted suicide that 'even if they got into a state where they were very dependent and felt very helpless and useless, their life was still precious ... Who knows what good things can come out of the last phase of a person's life?'

But Deborah Annetts, of Dignity in Dying, countered that had Lord Joffe's bill been in place, Anne Turner would not have had to take her life early – that she was forced to leave Britain while she was still able to travel. If the bill had been in place, she said, perhaps Anne Turner would still be alive.

It is clear that it will be many years before this controversy is settled. It is also clear that those who thought that putting Jack Kevorkian behind bars would settle the issue, that those who saw him as a villain, a man alone who wished to hasten people's journeys out of this life, were dead wrong. His wish, which was to help people end their suffering, is now part of a worldwide public debate. Whether or not assisted suicide is legalised in America, Great Britain or anywhere else in the world, Jack Kevorkian shone a spotlight on pain and suffering and because of him, the medical community has at last begun to pay attention to palliative care and the needs of the dying.

Unfortunately, 'Dr Death' has had to pay a steep price for this. Compare his sentence of 10 to 25 years in prison with that of Carol Carr, who in 2002 was convicted of assisting the suicide of her two grown sons, Andy and Rand, who were suffering from advanced stages of Huntington's Disease. Carr had watched her husband's slow death from the incurable disease and had made a suicide pact with her two sons, promising she would not let them suffer the same fate. So she took a gun into the Georgia nursing home where the boys were living and shot and killed them as they lay in their beds. Carr was sentenced to serve five years in prison, and was paroled after 21 months. Jack Kevorkian, convicted in 1999, will have been in prison for nine years before he is even eligible for parole. Perhaps Terry Youk, Tom Youk's brother, said it best when he described his feelings about Dr Kevorkian:

> This man is not a criminal, my brother is not a victim. Generations to come will scarce believe that Jack Kevorkian, MD, was villainized for acting in good conscience from his heart – in the process challenging the short sighted and putting his own life on the line for a simple choice.

I Shall Not Live in Vain

If I can stop one heart from breaking,
I shall not live in vain;
If I can ease one life the aching,
Or cool one pain,
Or help one fainting robin
Unto his nest again,
I shall not live in vain.

Emily Dickinson

About the Authors

Neal Nicol has been a friend and co-worker of Dr Jack Kevorkian since 1961. A laboratory technician and president of supply company Scientific Specialties, Inc, Neal's work with Kevorkian led to his arrest on two occasions. Now retired, Neal regularly visits Kevorkian in prison and continues to be a steadfast supporter of the right to die.

Harry Wylie has been a long-time friend and confidant of Dr Jack Kevorkian. While they often argued over some of Kervorkian's opinions and actions, their friendship has stood strong. Harry and his wife Arlene have visited Kevorkian on a monthly basis during his incarceration.